For EU product safety concerns:
IN TECH d.o.o., Prolaz Marije Krucifikse Kozulić 3, 51000 Rijeka, Croatia,
info@intechopen.com or visit our website at intechopen.com.

NEONATAL CARE

Edited by **Deborah Raines** and **Zoe Iliodromiti**

Neonatal Care
Edited by Deborah Raines and Zoe Iliodromiti

Published by InTech
Janeza Trdine 9, 51000 Rijeka, Croatia

Publishing Process Manager Marija Radja

Technical Editor Teodora Smiljanic

Cover Designer InTech Design Team

Additional hard copies can be obtained from orders@intechopen.com

Neonatal Care, Edited by Deborah Raines and Zoe Iliodromiti
p. cm.
ISBN 978-953-51-0692-0

Meet the editors

Dr Deborah Raines is a perinatal researcher, curriculum design consultant and educational technologist. She is currently working on a variety of projects designing and implementing innovative education and evidence based clinical programs. She is a Sigma Theta Tau International nursing expert for Sharecare.com. In addition, she is a methodologist and mentor for doctoral students. In 2012 Dr. Raines was appointed the editor of the Evidence Based Research column for Neonatal Network: The Journal of Neonatal Nursing.

Dr Zoe Iliodromiti completed Pediatrics training in Greece, 1999. Completed thesis, "Nitric oxide and regulation of airways smooth muscle function ", at Thessaly University Medical School, Larissa, Greece 2000. Currently works as Lecturer in Pediatrics and Neonatology, at Aretaieio Hospital, Medical School University of Athens, Athens, Greece. Has 20+ publications in peer-reviewed journals; wrote 2 books; 3 chapters in books; over 30 presentations at national and international meetings. Her research has been awarded and is mainly focused on the fetal and neonatal inflammation and diabetes.

Contents

Preface

Neonatology is evolving rapidly and finds itself today at the forefront of numerous developments. The aim of this book is to present updated clinical and experimental data in the area of Neonatology. The articles of this volume have been expressly included with the aim of deepening scientific understanding of the pathogenetic mechanisms implicated in neonatal disorders and of further motivating research by acquainting the reader with the current knowledge and future perspectives. The field of Neonatology is especially exacting given that the wishes and expectations of parents are very specific. This multi-author book includes seven Chapters embracing a particularly interesting selection of neonatal issues. We thus believe that it will be of considerable value to all healthcare professionals working within Neonatology, from the undergraduate medical student to the specialist doctor trainee, the senior neonatologist and the specialist nurse.

Chapter 1 of this book offers, with the use of logistic and ordered logistic regression models, a highly informative epidemiological study analyzing the association between low birthweight, one of the key reproductive health indicators, and multiple factors such as the geographical area of residence, the gender of the child, multiple births, the age and the educational status of the mother. A notable finding has been that mothers who had secondary education or higher were significantly and inversely associated with having babies of low birthweight. Additional essential information is presented in the study in Chapter 2 in which the main principles of an effective, evidence-based newborn care program are detailed. Delays in recognition of perinatal problems and in the decision to seek care for these problems, or tardiness in reaching a health facility that has the opportunity to offer quality care are discussed as they can lead to increased perinatal morbidity and mortality rates.

The third Chapter examines the effect of aggressive parenteral nutrition, defined as relatively high amounts of parenteral protein and lipid commencing on the first day of life in the occurrence of ex-utero growth retardation and associated morbidities. Also discussed are new effective therapies for necrotizing enterocolitis, short-gut syndrome, gastroschisis and neonatal hemochromatosis based on the synchronous principles of Neonatal Gastroenterology and Nutrition Care.

In Chapter 4 the controversial issue of the potential pathogenetic mechanisms of brain injury in preterm infants as well as the pathological aspects of this condition are presented. This Chapter moreover includes short discussion about recent research studies which seek to develop therapies targeting astrocytes, activated microglia and glutamate inhibition. The following article, Chapter 5, analyzes two of the most common manifestations of brain injury in premature infants: periventricular leukomalacia and intraventricular hemorrhage. Additionally, the results of an original prospective cohort study in Chile analyzing the pathologic findings in cases of brain injury in neonates of 32 weeks or less (or birth weight of 1500 or less) are presented. Chapter 6 examines the association between meconium stained amniotic fluid—in both term and premature infants—and fetal brain injury that could lead to an adverse neurodevelopmental outcome. The potential pathogenetic pathways of brain injury due to meconium stained amniotic fluid are analyzed, as it appears evident that fetal-neonatal brain injury is the common origin for severe neurological handicaps, such as cerebral palsy and mental retardation, usually diagnosed years after birth and more frequently in children born through meconium stained amniotic fluid.

Finally, Chapter 7 deals with one of the major problems in neonatal care, the presence of sleep apnea in premature infants. The main clinical features of apnea for its clinical diagnosis and therapy are analyzed, in combination with an interesting presentation of the process of sleep development from fetal to neonatal age, with the focus on respiratory alterations, such as apnea.

I would like to extend my warm thanks to the authors who kindly agreed to make important contributions to this book and also to convey my gratitude to them for expending so much time and endeavor to do so. I additionally cordially thank the team at InTech for their most valuable expert assistance in the creation of this work. Last but certainly not least, the other authors and I express our sincere hope that this book will fully satisfy and fulfill our readers' expectations and needs.

Zoe Iliodromiti, MD
Lecturer in Pediatrics and Neonatology
University of Athens Medical School
Aretaieio Hospital
Athens
Greece

1

Maternal Socio-Economic Status and Childhood Birth Weight: A Health Survey in Ghana

Edward Nketiah-Amponsah[1,*], Aaron Abuosi[2] and Eric Arthur[1]
[1]*Department of Economics, University of Ghana,*
[2]*Department of Public Administration and Health Services Management, University of Ghana, Ghana*

1. Introduction

Low birth weight (LBW) is one of the key reproductive health indicators whose outcome is influenced by consumption of reproductive health care. Rosenzweig and Schultz (1983) argue that one of the key measures of child health is that of birth weight. Birth weight is a good gauge of health of the child in the womb because the weight is taken immediately after birth. Consequently, a malnourished fetus will be born at low birth weight. On average, the worldwide incidence of low birth weight varies among countries, ranging from 4% to 6% in western countries like Sweden, France, United States and Canada (UNICEF 2003). Nevertheless, LBW is prevalent in developing countries especially those in the Sub-Saharan region due to the high levels of malnutrition and infectious diseases. A child's birth weight is an important indicator of the child's vulnerability to the risk of childhood illnesses and the chances of survival. Sub-Saharan Africa (SSA) has the second highest incidence of low birth weight infants the world over (16%), with South Central Asia being the highest at 27% (UNICEF and WHO 2004). The most recent evidence on Ghana shows that approximately 10% of all births are LBW (GSS, 2009). In particular, the UN envisages a reduction of low birth weight by at least one-third in the proportion of infants. This target is in fact, one of the seven major goals for the current decade of the "A World Fit for Children" programme of the United Nations (UN, 2004).

LBW is considered a major public health concern. Hence, a significant reduction in LBW is regarded as an important catalyst towards the achievement of the Millennium Development Goals (MDGs). LBW is defined as a birth weight of less than 2.5kg or 2500 grams. There are two types of LBW infants, that is, small-for-date and pre-term babies. Small-for-date infants are those who are delivered after a full gestation period of 37-40 weeks but due to intra-uterine growth retardation (IUGR), their birth weights are below 2.5 kg. Conversely, LBW can be caused by short gestation duration; <37 weeks of gestation as in the case of pre-term babies. LBW is immensely connected with fetal and neonatal morbidity and mortality

* Corresponding Author

(McCormick, 1985; Gortmaker and Wise, 1997; Caulfield et al. 2004). It is also a potential recipe for impaired cognitive development and the advent of chronic diseases in later life including diabetes and coronary heart disease (Bale et al. 2003). Other known triggers of LBW include maternal malnutrition, biological conditions such as multiple births, sex of the child, malaria episodes during pregnancy, complicated pregnancy due to pre-eclampsia or antepartum haemorrhage and behavioural or life style factors such as smoking (Vahdaninia, et al. 2008; Alderman and Behrman 2006; Bhargava et al. 2004). The literature on low birth weight on the African continent is on the ascendancy (see Mwabu 2008; Okurut 2009). In Botswana, Ubomba-Jaswa and Ubomba-Jaswa (1996) found that multiple births, birth order (first order), marital status and mothers' stature were important predictors for low birth weight. A study by Vahdaninia (2008) reports that primary and secondary education and non-smokers are highly correlated with low birth weights.

In the 2003 Ghana Demographic and Health Survey, information on birth weights is known for only 28% of babies born five years preceding the survey. In the 2008 GDHS however, birth weights were reported for 43 percent of births in the five years preceding the Survey, indicating a 15 percentage point improvement in birth weight registration as compared to the GDHS 2003. Generally, the low registration of birth weights is due to the high non-institutional and non-supervised deliveries mostly in the rural areas of the country[1]. Since many respondents did not deliver in health facilities and would not have had their babies weighed at birth, the survey solicited information on the women's own subjective assessment of whether their babies were average or larger than average, smaller than average or very small at birth (see Blanc and Wardlaw, 2004). Even though the mothers' reportage of the size of the infant is subjective, it can be a useful proxy for the weight of the child. Hence, this paper attempts to estimate the factors that influence the weight of a baby at birth using the sub-set of children who were actually weighed by the health facilities in addition to those whose weights are subjectively reported by their mothers. The novelty of this paper lies in the attempt to empirically estimate maternal socio-economic and demographic factors and perceived baby size at birth. Modelling mothers' evaluation of baby size at birth is an important step in solving the sample selection bias in reported birth weights due to low institutional delivery in developing countries such as Ghana (Okurut 2009 and Nwabu, 2008). To the best of our knowledge, this gap has not been explored since studies surveyed by far are entirely based on children who were actually weighed at birth at the health facilities. The study emphasises maternal attributes on infant birth weight due to the fact that birth weight is correlated between half siblings of the same mother but not of the same father because of the greater contribution of the maternal genotype and environment (Gluckman, 1994 and Walton, 1954). Among the socio-economic factors of interest are income (wealth), education, occupation or employment and marital status.

2. Related literature

Previous studies on the phenomenon in Ghana and elsewhere had paid less attention to mothers' subjective evaluation of the size of the baby. In the context of developing countries where institutional delivery is very low, concentrating only on the children weighed at the health facilities creates some informational gap. The effects of socio-economic, biological

---

[1] Approximately, 57% of deliveries occur in health facilities, with the public health facilities accounting for 46% of such deliveries.

and nutritional attributes of LBW are well documented (Klufio et. al. 2000; Dreyfuss et al. 2001). The key determinants of birth weight include nutritional status and age of the mother, area of residence, mother's immunization against preventable diseases and behavioural change during pregnancy (Deshmukh et al. 1998; Stephenson and Symons, 2002; UNICEF, 2003; Torres-Arreola et al. 2005; Negi, et al. 2006, Khatun and Rahman, 2008).

Utilization of maternal health services such as immunization against tetanus is further assumed to be complementary to other inputs that improve the health of the child in the womb, such as presumptive malaria treatment and avoidance of risky behaviours (Dow et al, 1999). Ajakaiye and Mwabu (2007) argue that tetanus vaccination does not directly increase birth weight, but that vaccination is strongly correlated with health care consumption and behaviours that increase birth weight implication; the adoption of a specific behaviour or the uptake of a specific input improves health, creates incentives to engage in other health-augmenting behaviours or consumption that improve birth weight. Guyatt and Snow (2004) also argue that that malaria infection have a substantial adverse effect on pregnancy outcomes (causing both premature birth [gestation of <37weeks] and intrauterine growth retardation, which lead to LBW).

Employing the 2006 Uganda Demographic and Health Survey (UDHS) data, 2006, Bategeka et al. (2009) examined the factors that influence birth weight in Uganda using instrumental variable (2SLS) technique. The findings suggest that birth weight is positively and significantly influenced by the mother's tetanus immunization status, education level, and antenatal care, but negatively influenced by mother's smoking of tobacco and malaria infection. In a related study, Okurut (2009) investigated the determinants of birth weight in Botswana. Applying instrumental variable (2SLS) technique to the Botswana Family Health Survey (BFHS) data for 1996, he found that birth weight is positively and significantly influenced by the mother's socio-economic characteristics (tetanus immunization status, age, and education level) and the husband's education level. The results from Bategeka (2006) and Okurut (2009) reinforce the role of maternal socio-economic factors and biomedical inputs such as antenatal care services and tetanus vaccination on childhood birth weight. The authors thus suggested that policy should be geared at, improving education of the girl child and improving access to reproductive health services (tetanus immunization and quality antenatal care) is critical in enhancing the health status of the unborn children in Botswana.

Similar evidence was adduced by Deshmukh (1998) who noted that tobacco exposure was a significant risk factor for LBW. Further empirical evidence by Almond et al (2002) also suggested that maternal smoking during pregnancy has negative and significant effects on birth weight and gestation length. Mwabu (2008) and Okurut (2009) sought to identify the determinants of birth weight in Kenya and Botswana respectively. In both studies, a two-stage least squares approach was adopted and the results were comparable. The mother's characteristics, age, education level and tetanus immunization were found to have a positive significant impact on birth weight. In both studies, tetanus immunization was used as an instrument for antenatal visits.

This paper uses the most recent nationally representative Demographic and Health Survey, GDHS 2008 to throw more light on the factors that contribute to the relatively high prevalence of low birth weight in Ghana. Contrary to most studies where birth weight is modelled as a continuous variable, this study measures birth weight as a discrete outcome.

3. Overview of the Ghanaian health sector

Prior to Ghana's independence from the British crown, the colonial administration provided healthcare for civil servants through general taxation while non-civil servants received healthcare at their own expense (out-of-pocket). Following Ghana's independence in 1957, health care was provided "freely" to subscribers of public health facilities. This ensured that there was no direct out-of-pocket payment at the point of delivery of health care in public health facilities. Financing of health in the public sector was, therefore, entirely through tax revenues. The sustainability of the free medical care policy became questionable as the economy began to show signs of decline in the 1970s and 1980s with economic growth and inflation being the major culprits. The ensuing economic decline eventually ushered Ghana into the World Bank/IMF's sponsored ERP/Structural Adjustment Programmes during the 1980s and 1990s. A key component of the ERP was health sector reform, which was intended to improve the efficiency of the health systems and the quality of care via cost recovery mechanism, in particular out-of-pocket payments with its concomitant effect of decreasing access to health care by the poor (Nyonator and Kutzin, 1999; Asenso-Okyere et al, 1997).

Consequently, Ghana has since 1985, operated a cost-recovery health delivery system known as the "cash-and-carry" system, whereby patients are required to pay up-front for health services at government clinics and hospitals. The advent of out-of-pocket payments constrained access to health care to many Ghanaians especially during emergency and accident cases where deposits are required before care. This coupled with reduction in public spending on health care created problems of inaccessibility and inequity in health care.

In the midst of these financing challenges, the Government of Ghana and its global partners consider the improvement of maternal health as crucial for socio-economic development. In 1987, the World Health Organization (WHO) and other UN agencies including UNICEF launched the Safe Motherhood Initiative which was genially embraced by Ghana. In 1998, the government introduced a free antenatal care services for all pregnant women. The commitment of the government of Ghana in promoting safe motherhood was further enhanced by the introduction of the policy of exempting users of maternal services from delivery fees in the four most deprived regions of Ghana namely, Upper East, Upper West, Northern and Central, in September 2003. The policy was later expanded to incorporate the remaining six regions of Ghana in April 2005. Furthermore, the government of Ghana armed with a grant support of US$90 million from the UK government in July 2008 strengthened the free maternal care initiative (Government of Ghana, 2010, United Nations, 2008). The main rationale for the introduction of these policies is to reduce financial barriers and to induce the utilization of maternal health services with the overall objective of improving maternal and child health outcomes including birth weight. Other policies introduced by the government to improve access and equity to essential health care services include the introduction of interventions such as the Community-based Health Planning and Services (CHPS) and the introduction of the National Health Insurance Scheme (NHIS) and the free maternal care programme. However, access still remains a problem. For instance, institutional delivery remains a low of 53% (WHO, 2011).

Country	LBW	IMR	U5MR	MI	MMR	LE	PCHE
Ghana	**14.3**	**47**	**69**	**93**	**350**	**60**	**114**
Nigeria	26.7	86	138	41	840	54	113
Benin	20.2	75	118	72	410	57	61
Burkina Faso	37.4	91	166	75	560	52	82
Cape Verde	-	23	27	96	94	71	176
Cote D'Ivoire	16.7	83	118	67	470	50	88
Gambia	15.8	78	103	96	400	60	75
Guinea Conakry	20.8	88	142	51	680	52	58
Liberia	20.4	80	112	64	990	56	46
Mali	27.9	101	191	71	830	53	76
Niger	39.9	76	160	73	820	57	40
Senegal	14.5	51	93	79	410	62	102
Sierra Leone	21.3	123	192	71	970	49	104
Togo	20.5	64	98	84	350	59	70
Guinea Bissau	17.4	115	193	76	1000	49	48
African Average	-	80	127	69	620	54	146

Table 1. Selected Health Indicators for Ghana and other Regional Neighbours (ECOWAS). LBW=Low Birth weight; IMR=Infant Mortality Rate; MI=Measles Immunization; MMR=Maternal Mortality Rate; LE=Life Expectancy; PCHE= Per capita Health Expenditure. *Source: World Health Statistics 2011. World Health Organization, Geneva*

The passage of the National Health Insurance law in 2003 (Government of Ghana, 2003) was in particular to remove the financial barrier to health care and to promote access and equity. The Act mandates the establishment of District-wide mutual health insurance schemes (DMHIS) where minimum premium of roughly US$8 per adult (Jehu-Appiah et al. 2011) for non Social Security and National insurance trust contributors are charged. The scheme provides generous exemptions for those aged under 18, and over 70, pensioners, pregnant women or deemed indigent (core poor). Formal and informal sector employees who contribute to the Social Security and National Insurance Trust (SSNIT) pay 2.5% of their SSNIT contributions as insurance premium. Though enrolment is compulsory, non-compliance is quite high while there are virtually no enforcement mechanisms.

While Ghana's selected health indicators are better than almost all its West African neighbours, the indicators do not compare favourably with other countries within the African sub-region, with the gap widening in comparison with the developed world (see Table 1 and WHO Health Reports, 2010 and 2011). Migration of health workforce, inadequate health personnel (high doctor patient ratio), poor health infrastructure and general dissatisfaction with working conditions are some of the major challenges facing the country's health sector (Ghana Health Service, 2007; Agyepong *et al.* 2004)

4. Methods

4.1 Data

The study uses the 2008 Ghana Demographic and Health Survey (GDHS), the fifth Demographic and Health Survey (DHS) to be undertaken in Ghana since 1988. It is a nationally representative household survey conducted by the Ghana Statistical Service with technical support from the World Bank. The 2008 GDHS was implemented in a representative probability sample of more than 12,000 households selected throughout Ghana. The survey centred on general welfare, education, health and healthcare and demographic issues that impinge on the wellbeing of women, children and the average Ghanaian household. Three questionnaires were used for the 2008 GDHS: (i) the Household Questionnaire, (ii) the Women's Questionnaire, and (iii) the Men's Questionnaire. In all, 4,916 women aged 15-49 and 4,568 men aged 15-59 from 6,141 households were interviewed from all the ten regions of Ghana from early September to late November 2008. This study is based on the maternal questionnaire which contains detailed information on fertility, marriage, sexual activity, fertility preferences, breastfeeding practices, nutritional status of women and young children and other socioeconomic attributes of the women. The study sample consists of children who were born within the five years preceding the 2007-08 GDHS and whose mothers were interviewed in the survey. The analyses will thus be based on children aged 0-59 months who were weighed at birth and those whose mothers subjectively reported their size at birth. The variables which were included in the empirical estimation are shown in Table 2.

5. Estimation

In this paper, the birth weight of the infant is captured as a dichotomous and in an ordered form. In the case of the dichotomous dependent variable, cases with a birth weight of below 2.5 kg (2500grams) are considered LBW while those with 2.5kg or more are non-LBW. With regards to the ordered birth size, the mothers' subjective assessment of their babies is ranked from very large, the highest which is accorded a value of one(1) to very small, the lowest which is assigned a value of five (5) with 5 categories as presented in Table 3. Discrete choice, particularly the logistic and ordered logistic regressions are used to estimate the correlates of low birth weight. The use of these methods is appropriate and enables us to assess each explanatory variable with the likelihood of a child having low birth weight. Where appropriate the marginal effects and/or the odds ratios are computed to ease the interpretation.

5.1 Logit

The Logistic model is used for the prediction of the probability of occurrence of a discrete binary variable. It is employed in cases where the variable has only two outcomes. As employed in this study, the outcome variable is coded zero(0) if the child has normal weight(>=2500grams) and coded one (1) if the baby weighs below 2500grams in which case the child is considered to have low birth weight. Gujarati (2004) estimates the logistic regression model as;

$$Y^* = \beta_0 + \sum_{i=1}^{k} \beta_i X_i + e_i$$

Where;

Y* = Dependent variable (Birth weight)
X_i = Independent variables; maternal bio-demographic and socioeconomic characteristics
β_0 = Intercept
β_i = Regression coefficients

The model is estimated using Stata.

5.2 Ordered logit

The ordered logistic model is a regression model for ordinal dependent variables. It is an extension of the logistic regression model for binary dependent variables, allowing for more than two ordered response categories. It is usually estimated using the maximum likelihood estimation technique. The ordered logistic model, according to Greene (2003) can be written as,

$$y_i^* = \beta' x_i + \varepsilon .$$

Where y_i^* = the underlying response, which is the birth weight of the baby.

x_i = a set of explanatory variables and u_i = the residual error, which is assumed to be normally distributed.

According to Greene (2003), y*, the variable of interest (which is the subjective or perceived birth weight of the baby) is unobserved, what we observe rather is a variable y, which in this study is the size of the baby as ranked by the mother. Consequently, we model the mother's perceived size of the baby at birth using a 5 point Likert scale from very large (1), larger than average (2), average (3), smaller than average (4) and very small (5) where very large (1) is the highest and very small (5) is the lowest.

5.3 Results and discussion

5.4 Logistic regression

The mean birth weight for the entire sample is 3239.24 grams (SD=832.30) while the mean birth weights for the normal and LBW infants are 3368.0 (SD=761.99) and 2098.90(SD=302.11) grams respectively. At the bivariate level, gender and multiple births were significantly different between mothers of LBW and normal birth weight infants (see Table 2). Multivariate analysis however, showed that multiple birth (odds ratio = 13.72) was the most important risk factor for LBW in Ghana.

The wealth index of the household (used as a proxy for household income) was constructed in quintiles (1 = poorest, 2 = poorer, 3 = middle, 4 = richer, 5= richest). The results suggest that women in the poorest wealth quintile are less likely to have LBW compared to those in the highest income quintiles, though this was only significant at the 10% (p = *0.065*). However, those in the poorer, middle and richer quintiles did not show significant association with LBW. Our finding is in sharp contrast with that of Torres-Arreola et al. (2005) who found low socio-economic status as the most important risk factor for

LBW.Though this result is not unexpected, it is not inexplicable. The wealth index is used a proxy for income since there is no direct measure of income. Wealth per se is not a direct determinant of health outcome unless it is translated into the consumption of health inputs. We can thus conclude that we did not detect any significant relationship between wealth index and LBW for Ghana. Normally, differences found in the effect of socioeconomic factors on LBW are probably due to the use of different socioeconomic indicators. It should be noted however, that obtaining information that accurately reflects social and economic characteristics can be difficult, leading to the generation of proxy variables.

Education as expected proved significant in explaining LBW in Ghana. Our finding indicates that there is a threshold effect of education on LBW. While primary education has the expected negative relationship, it is statistically insignificant. Rather, it is secondary education or better which exerts the requisite effect on LBW. In particularly, women who have secondary education or better are 6 percentage points less likely to have LBW compared to their counterparts with no education. The significant inverse relationship between education and LBW is consistent with Koupilova et al. (2000), Mwabu (2008), Khatun and Rahman (2008) and Okurut (2009). Although other studies have reported the negative effect of maternal education on LBW, the association was not statistically significant (see Torres-Arreola et al. 2005; Ubomba-Jaswa and-Ubomba-Jaswa, 1996). In Iran, Jafari et al. (2010) rather found a positive and significant relationship between primary and secondary education on one hand and LBW on the other hand. The results also indicate that the gender of the child is highly associated with birth weight. A boy child has a higher probability of experiencing low birth weight relative to a girl child. More specifically, being a boy increases the odds of LBW by 1.7 (3 percentage points) relative to their girl counterparts.

The study's finding further points to a significant regional variation in low birth weights. Women in the Western region (p=0.005), Ashanti(p=0.042) and the Brong-Ahafo (p=0.090) have a higher propensity of giving birth to LBWs as compared to children born in the Greater Accra Region. For instance, children born to women in the western region of Ghana are approximately 16 percentage points more likely to be of LBW compared to their counterparts in the Greater Accra region. The descriptive statistics in Table 2 also lend support to this empirical finding. Although women who are employed showed the expected inverse relationship with LBW, the effect is insignificant.

Variable : Birth weight	**Normal birth weight**	**Low birth weight**	**Pearson's chi square test**
Wealth			
poorest	96.94	3.06	5.36
poorer	90.32	9.68	
middle	89.76	10.24	
richer	90.64	9.36	
richest	92.73	7.27	
Education			
no education	91.86	8.14	
primary	90.34	9.66	
secondary	92.02	7.98	
Mother's Age			
15 - 19 years	97.06	2.94	2.29
20 - 34 years	91.99	8.01	

Variable : Birth weight	Normal birth weight	Low birth weight	Pearson's chi square test
35 - 49 years	89.91	10.09	
Tetanus Injection			
No injections	94.12	5.88	0.59
Received Injections	91.44	8.56	
Birth order			
1 child	93.01	6.99	0.94
2 - 5 children	91.44	8.56	
More than 5 children	90.36	9.64	
Gender of Child			
Male	93.36	6.64	3.60*
Female	89.81	10.19	
Birth type			
Single birth	92.57	7.43	31.74***
Multiple birth	61.54	38.46	
ANC			
No visits	87.5	12.5	0.65
1 - 3 visits	89.77	10.23	
4 or more visits	91.9	8.1	
Rural*Education			
No education	92.47	7.53	2.28
Primary	91.76	8.24	
Secondary plus	89.01	10.99	
Residence			
Urban	92.46	7.54	0.98
Rural	90.6	9.4	
Employment			
Not working	93.55	6.45	0.68
Working	91.33	8.67	
Marital status			
Not married	91.67	8.33	0.0001
Married	91.65	8.35	
Administrative Regions			
Western	84.93	15.07	12.83
Central	92.86	7.14	
Greater Accra	95.51	4.49	
Volta	91.67	8.33	
Eastern	89.8	10.2	
Ashanti	89.52	10.48	
Brong Ahafo	90.41	9.59	
Northern	94.74	5.26	
Upper East	98	2	
Upper West	91.67	8.33	

Tables 2. Bivariate Analysis for Selected Variables 2008[2]. ***: Significant at 1 %($p<0.001$); **: Significant at 5% ($p<0.05$ and *: Significant at 10% ($p<0.10$)

[2] The variables for the empirical estimation were chosen with recourse to the literature and the peculiarity of the health care situation of a developing country. For instance, alcohol consumption and

The age of the woman is hypothesized to be statistically and significantly associated with LBW overtime. This variable is statistically significant at the 10% level. That is, an increase in the age of an expectant mother by one year increases the probability of giving birth to a LBW by 3 percentage points. The positive association between maternal age and LWB which is largely due to the health depreciation effect is consistent with Vahdaninia et al.(2008) Who found same for Iran. Further, women who live in the urban areas have a lower propensity of giving birth to LBWs but this variable is not significant.

Dependent Variable : Birth weight	**Coefficient**	**Standard**	**P>z**	**Marginal Effects**	**Odds Ratio**
Wealth (Ref: Richest)					
Poorest	-1.506*	0.816	0.065	-0.055	0.222
Poorer	-0.31	0.484	0.521	-0.016	0.733
Middle	-0.045	0.462	0.923	-0.003	0.956
Richer	0.045	0.374	0.905	0.003	1.046
Mother's Education					
Primary	-0.386	0.464	0.406	-0.02	0.68
Secondary plus	-0.944**	0.482	0.05	-0.06	0.389
Other Socioeconomic Indicators					
Mother's Age	0.583*	0.337	0.083	0.033	1.791
Tetanus Injecton given	-0.672	0.549	0.221	-0.03	0.511
Multiple birth	2.619***	0.47	0	0.395	13.718
Gender of child: Female	0.524**	0.266	0.049	0.03	1.689
Rural and Educated	0.406	0.355	0.252	0.023	1.501
Mother's Body mass index	0.0001	0	0.738	0	1
Antenatal care visits	-0.109	0.133	0.416	-0.006	0.897
Birth Order	-0.149*	0.084	0.076	-0.009	0.861
Residence: Rural	-0.034	0.576	0.953	-0.002	0.967
Employment (Ref: Not working)	-0.132	0.433	0.761	-0.007	0.877
Marital status(Ref: Not married)	-0.219	0.419	0.6	-0.014	0.803
Administrative Regions					
Western	1.539**	0.548	0.005	0.156	4.658
Central	0.423	0.773	0.585	0.029	1.526
Volta	0.669	0.711	0.347	0.05	1.952
Eastern	0.842	0.547	0.124	0.065	2.32
Ashanti	1.028**	0.506	0.042	0.076	2.794
Brong Ahafo	0.988*	0.582	0.09	0.082	2.685
Northern	0.031	0.717	0.966	0.002	1.031
Upper East	-0.555	1.171	0.636	-0.026	0.574
Upper West	0.955	0.708	0.177	0.08	2.599
Constant	-3.382	1.238	0.006		
Number of observations : 874	LR chi2(26) = 55.07		Prob>chi2 = 0.0007		
Log likelihood = -223.56078	Pseudo R2 = 0.1097				

Table 3. Logit estimates of the effects of maternal socio-economic factors and LBW. ***: Significant at 1 %(p<0.001); **: Significant at 5% (p<0.05 and *: Significant at 10% (p<0.10)

---

cigarette smoking were not included because only few women indicated the use of alcohol and smoking of cigarette during pregnancy. The inclusion of these variables would create a problem of matrix singularity.

The results also indicate a negative association between LBW and the number of antenatal care visits, though the effect is not robust. Antenatal care visits are used to diagnose and treat for any infections which affect the unborn babies. The results suggest that the higher the number of antenatal visits, the lower the probability of LBW. Other studies including Negi et al (2006) and Joshi et al (2005) had found a significant negative correlation between mother's antenatal care visits and LBW.

The most robust finding from our study is the significant statistical relationship between multiple births and LBW ($p<0.0001$). Children who are born twins or mutilple are approximately 40 percentage points more likely to be of LBW as compared to singletons. This finding is consistent with Ubomba-Jaswa and Ubomba-Jaswa (1996) who found a robust positive association between multiple births and LBW for infants in Botswana. Thus, if women who had not received immunization against tetanus were to be immunized, the probability of experiencing a LBW will drop by 3 percentage points. The low birth weight of twins compared with singletons is somewhat influenced by the higher congenital abnormality rate in twins, or the increased incidence of proteinuric pre-eclampsia in the mothers, (MacGillivray, 1983). Also, vaccination against tetanus was found to have the desired negative effect on LBW, albeit insignificant ($p=0.221$). We also found an inverse relationship between birth order and LBW. Our finding is however at variance with Phung et al. (2003) who found that higher parity was associated with significantly higher birth weight.

5.5 Ordered logistic regression

At the bivariate level (see Table 4), the Pearson chi-square test indicates that there are statistically significant differences between perceived birth size on one hand and the gender of the child, antenatal care visits, marital status, area of residence and geographical area of residence on the other hand ($p<0.001$). However, a number of covariates contemporaneously determine an outcome such as birth weight, hence the result from the multivariate ordered logistic regression is emphasized.

Variable : child size at birth	Very large (1)	Larger than Average (2)	Average (3)	Smaller than average (4)	Very small (5)	Pearson's chi square test
Wealth						
Poorest	20.3	32.01	29.37	12.54	5.78	23.65*
Poorer	24.29	31.07	31.51	8.97	4.16	
Middle	22.74	32.33	33.7	6.85	4.38	
Richer	20.9	34.39	32.54	8.73	3.44	
Richest	24.15	37.74	25.66	9.81	2.64	
Education						
No education	23.71	31.98	28.73	10.57	5.01	11.66
Primary	19.43	31.58	33.2	11.13	4.66	
Secondary	22.53	34.8	30.99	8.1	3.58	
Gender of child						
Male	255	364	330	81	35	19.52***
Female	20.38	31.81	30.42	11.93	5.47	

Birth type						
Single birth	22.38	33.15	30.73	9.44	4.3	
Multiple	14.89	27.66	29.79	21.28	6.38	
Birth Order						
1	19.37	32.88	31.98	10.36	5.41	6.64
2	22.55	34.06	30.45	8.85	4.09	
3	23.78	31.25	30.21	10.76	3.99	
Antenatal Care						
No visits	17.07	24.39	36.59	9.76	12.2	21.28***
1 -3 visits	21.37	31.34	29.91	11.68	5.7	
4 or more visits	22.65	33.82	30.59	9.28	3.66	
Employment						
Not working	22.35	32.95	30.79	9.6	4.3	0.4
Working	21.24	33.59	30.12	10.42	4.63	
Married						
Not married	16.6	29.79	37.45	10.21	5.96	10.18**
Married	22.93	33.44	29.85	9.64	4.14	
Residence						
Urban	23.58	36.31	29.13	8.27	2.71	15.15***
Rural	21.46	31.21	31.58	10.5	5.25	
Rural* Education						
No Education	23.58	33.96	28.81	9.7	3.96	10.72
Primary	19.57	31.19	33.64	10.7	4.89	
Secondary plus	19.8	31.44	34.65	8.91	5.2	
Tetanus Injection						
No injection	20.78	30.59	31.37	9.41	7.84	13.18
Received Injections	22.39	33.43	30.56	9.76	3.86	
Mother's Age						
15 - 19 years	16.83	30.69	36.63	11.88	3.96	12.71
20 - 34 years	20.94	34.44	29.87	10.25	4.5	
35 - 49 years	25.9	30.29	31.6	8.14	4.07	
Region						
Western	18.38	28.65	46.49	5.41	1.08	239.62***
Central	22.73	32.47	38.31	5.84	0.65	
Greater Accra	20.4	44.28	25.37	8.46	1.49	
Volta	6.86	32.57	44.57	14.86	1.14	
Eastern	34.64	31.84	20.11	6.15	7.26	
Ashanti	22.29	28.66	35.67	6.05	7.32	
Brong Ahafo	9.9	41.09	33.66	11.88	3.47	
Northern	38.98	27.12	14.92	10.85	8.14	
Upper East	16.05	35.19	27.78	14.2	6.79	
Upper West	22.06	33.33	27.94	14.71	1.96	

Tables 4. Bivariate Analysis for the Variables used for the Ordered Logistic Regression (Mother's Perception of Baby Size). ***: Significant at 1 %(p<0.001); **: Significant at 5% (p<0.05 and *: Significant at 10% (p<0.10)

Variable : Birth size	Coefficients	Robust Standard Error	z	P>z
Wealth (Ref: Richest)				
Poorest	0.064	0.195	0.33	0.742
Poorer	-0.252	0.179	-1.41	0.159
Middle	-0.158	0.164	-0.96	0.336
richer	0.009	0.152	0.06	0.951
Mother's Education				
Primary	-0.05	0.143	-0.35	0.728
Secondary plus	-0.320*	0.178	-1.8	0.072
Other Socioeconomic Indicators				
Age	-0.08	0.102	-0.79	0.432
Tetanus injection	0.078	0.137	0.57	0.568
Multiple births	0.874***	0.283	3.09	0.002
Gender (female)	0.276***	0.081	3.42	0.001
Rural*Educated	0.134	0.107	1.26	0.209
BMI of mother	0.0001	0	-0.13	0.899
Antenatal care visits	-0.068**	0.036	-1.91	0.057
Birth order	-0.026	0.026	-0.99	0.324
Rural	0.097	0.175	0.56	0.579
Employment (not working)	0.07	0.124	0.57	0.57
Marital Status (not married)	-0.399***	0.134	-2.97	0.003
Administrative Regions	-	-	-	-
Western	0.263	0.174	1.51	0.131
Central	-0.033	0.191	-0.17	0.864
Volta	0.679***	0.173	3.92	0
Eastern	-0.416**	0.203	-2.05	0.041
Ashanti	0.289*	0.168	1.73	0.084
Brong Ahafo	0.422**	0.171	2.47	0.013
Northern	-0.503**	0.206	-2.44	0.015
Upper East	0.305	0.221	1.38	0.167
Upper West	0.073	0.195	0.37	0.71
Number of Observations: 2072 Wald chi2(26) = 138.73 Prob>chi2 = 0.000 Log pseudolikelihood = -2894.5102 Pseudo R^2 = 0.0223				

Table 5. Ordered Logit Estimates of the effects of Maternal Socio-economic Factors and Perceived Baby Size. ***: Significant at 1 %(p<0.001); **: Significant at 5% (p<0.05 and *: Significant at 10% (p<0.10)

Table 5, presents the results of the ordered logistic regression where the size of the baby is ranked from very large (1), lager than average (2), average (3), smaller than average (4) to very small (5). A negative value denotes a movement from a very small size at birth towards a very large size at birth while a positive suggests otherwise. None of the wealth indicators was found to statistically influence perceived size of the baby. Just as in the first model, the results suggest that mothers with secondary education or better are less likely to perceive LBW. Though, primary education had the a priori expectation, it was insignificant, buttressing the threshold effect of secondary education on childhood birth weight. Interestingly, we found that higher birth orders are associated with a lower risk of perceived LBW (*p=0.007*).

The gender of the child was another variable that was found to exert significant influence on perceived size of the baby (*p=0.001*). Children born males are more likely to gravitate from very large baby size towards very small baby size relative to their female counterparts. The gender difference in perceived size might be due to the differences in the biological attributes. The gender effect is corroborated by the estimations in Table 3 where males were found to have a higher probability of LBW. Also residents of the Western and Volta geographical regions of Ghana have a higher propensity of experiencing perceived LBW than those residing in the greater Accra region. However, women in the Northern region of Ghana are less likely to have LBW (*p=0.004*). This result is quite surprising given that the Northern region is one of the poorest regions of Ghana. It is, thus probable that some attributes inherent in the region other than wealth and the consumption of biomedical inputs promote perceived normal birth sizes.

Unlike the logistic regression model where LBW is predicted, the effect of marital status (*p=0.003*) and antenatal care visits (*p= 0.057*) are correctly signed and significant in predicting perceived baby size by mothers. More specifically, married women and those who intensify the use of antenatal care visits are less likely to register LBW. These variables were also found to be significant at the bivariate level (see Table 4). Other covariates including urban residence had no significant effect on perceived baby size while that of multiple births had a positive and significant association with same.

6. Summary and concluding remarks

In summary, LBW is positively and significantly predicted by geographical area of residence, gender of the child, multiple births and mother's age. Conversely, maternal education especially beyond the primary education and birth order were found to be statistically and inversely related to LBW. In particular, women with secondary education or better are approximately 39 percentage points less likely to experience LBW relative to their uneducated counterparts. While biomedical inputs such as immunization against tetanus and the number of antenatal care visits have the expected inverse relationship, they proved insignificant in predicting LBW.

The ordered logistic regression indicates that marital status, the utilization of antenatal care services, secondary education or better and residents of the Eastern and Northern geographical regions of Ghana are significantly and inversely associated LBW. However, multiple births, gender, and residents of Volta and Northern geographical regions are positively and significantly associated with having babies with small sizes. Overall, multiple births, gender and secondary education or better were consistently significant in predicting LBW and perceived baby size in both the logistic and ordered logistic regression models.

Although, the proxy for income (wealth index) did not prove to be an important determinant, other studies have used education as a proxy for socio-economic status (Nordstrom and Cnattingius, 1996; Parker et al. 1994). At least, using data from the most recent survey, we have demonstrated a strong inverse association between secondary education or better and LBW.

In the context of a free and universal access to health care, it is recommended that policy makers should place more emphasis on education as it imparts knowledge and thus influences dietary habits and birth-spacing behaviour. This will lead to a better nutritional status, particularly in dealing with pregnancy, resulting in lower rates of low birth weight. Thus the government should target policies that reduce the regional disparities in health facilities and infrastructure to curb the regional differences in birth weight outcomes. Due to the robust effect of education on health outcomes including birth weight, intensifying especially girl child education via formal and informal means in addition to the provision of health infrastructure constitutes an important policy intervention.

7. References

Alderman, H., and Behrman, J. (2006). "Reducing the Incidence of Low Birth Weight in Low-Income Countries Has Substantial Economic Benefits." *World Bank Research Observer*, 21(1):25-48.

Agyepong, I. A., Anafi, P., Asiamah, E., Ansah, E. K., Ashon, D. A., & Narh-Dometey, C. (2004). Health worker (internal customer) satisfaction and motivation in the public sector health care providers. *International Journal of Health Planning and Management*, 19(4):319-36.

Ajakaiye, O. and Mwabu, G. (2007). The Demand for Reproductive Health Services: An Application of Control Function Approach. AERC Working Paper Series.

Bale, J. R., Stoll, B.J., Lucas, A.O. (2003). (eds). Improving Birth Outcomes: Meeting the Challenge in the Developing World. Washington, D.C: The National Academies Press.

Bategeka, L., Leah, M., Okurut, A., Barungi, M., Apolot, J. M. (2009). The Determinants of Birth weight in Uganda. A Final Report Submitted to AERC, Nairobi, Kenya.

Bhargava, S.K., Sachdev, H.S., Fall, C. H .D, Osmond, C., Lakshmy, R., Barker, D. J. P., Biswas, S. K. D., Ramji, S., Prabhakaran, D. and Reddy, K. S. (2004). Relation of Serial Changes in Childhood Body-Mass Index to Impaired Glucose Tolerance in Young Adulthood. *New England Journal of Medicine*, 350:865-75.

Blanc, A. K. and Wardlaw, T. (2004). Monitoring Low Birth Weight: An Evaluation of International Estimates and an Update Estimation Procedure, *Bulletin of the World Health Organization*, 83:3.

Blunch, N. (2004), "Maternal Literacy and Numeracy Skills and Child Health in Ghana" A paper presented at the Northeast Universities Development Consortium Conference, HEC Montreal, October 1-3, 2004.

Caulfield, L. E., De Onis, M., Blossner, M., Black, R. E. (2004). Under nutrition as an Underlying Cause of child deaths associated with Diarrhoea, pneumonia, malaria and measles. *American Journal of Clinical Nutrition*, 80: 193-198.

Deshmukh, J.S,. Motghare, D. D. Zodpey, S. P and Wadhva, S.K. (1998). Low birth weight and associated maternal factors in an urban area, *Indian paediatrics*, 35: 33-36

Dreyfuss, M. L., Msamanga, G. I., Spiegelmam, D., Hunter, D. J., Ernest, Urassa, E. J. N., Hertzmark E. and Fawzi, W. W. (2001). Determinants of Low Birth Weight among HIV-infected Pregnant Women in Tanzania, American Journal of Clinical Nutrition, 74(6): 814-826.

Ghana Health Service. (2007). Annual report. Ministry of health, Accra. Ghana Statistical Service Ghana Statistical Service and Macro International Inc. (MI). (2004). Ghana Demographic and Health Survey 2003. Calverton, Maryland: GSS and MI.

Ghana Statistical Service (GSS) and Macro International Inc. (MI). (2009). Ghana Demographic and Health Survey 2008. Calverton, Maryland: GSS and MI.

Government of Ghana(GOG). The National Health Insurance Act: Act650. Accra: Government of Ghana.

Gortmaker, S. L., Wise, P. (1997). The First Injustice: Socio-economic Disparities, Health Services Technology and Infant Mortality. *Annual Review of Sociology*, 23:147-70

Gluckman, P, Harding J. E. (1994). Nutritional and hormonal regulation of fetal growth: evolving concepts. *Acta Paediatrica*(Suppl)399:60–3.

Jafari , F, Eftekhar, H, . Pourreza, A. and Mousavi, J. (2010). Socio-economic and medical determinants of low birth weight in Iran: 20 years after establishment of a primary healthcare network. *Public Health*, 124(3):153-158.

Jehu-Appiah, C., Aryeetey, G., Agyepong, I. Spaan, E. and Baltussen, R. (2011). Household Perceptions and their implications for enrolment in the National Health Insurance Scheme in Ghana. *Health Policy and Planning*, 2011:1-12. doi: 10.1093/heapol/czr032.

Joshi, H. S., Subba, S. H., Dabral1, S. B., Dwivedi, S., Kumar, D. and Singh, S. (2005). Risk Factors Associated with Low Birth Weight in Newborns. *Indian Journal of Community Medicine*, 30: 4.

Hernández, S., Villa-Barragán, Juan Pablo and Rendón-Macías, E (2005). Socioeconomic factors and low birth weight in Mexico. *BMC Public Health*, 5:20 .doi:10.1186/1471-2458-5-20.

Khatun, S. and Rahman, M. (2008). Socio-economic determinants of low birth weight in Bangladesh: a multivariate approach. *Bangladesh Medical Research Council Bulletin*. 34(3):81-6

Klufio, C. A., Lassey, A. T, Annan, B. D. and Wilson, J. B. (2000). Birth weight Distribution at Korle-Bu Teaching Hospital, Ghana. *East African Medical Journal*, 78(8):418-423.

Koupilova, I, Rahu, Kaja, Rahu, M,, Karro, H. and Leon, D. A. (2000). Social determinants of birth weight and length of gestation in Estonia during the transition to democracy, *International Journal of Epidemiology*, 29:118–124

MacGillivray, I. (1983). Determinants of birth weight of twins. *Acta Genet Med Gemellol* (Roma).32(2):151-7

McCormick, M.C. (1985). The Contribution of Low Birth Weight to Infant Mortality and Childhood Morbidity, *New England Journal of Medicine.* 312: 82-90.

Mbuya, M. N. N., Children, M., Chasekwa, B. and Mishra, V. (2010). Biological, Social and Environmental Determinants of Low Birth Weight and Stunting among Infants and Young Children in Zimbabwe, Zimbabwe Working Papers, No.7.

Negi, K.S., Kandpal, S.D. and Kukreti, M. (2006), "Epidemiological Factors Affecting Low Birth Weight", *JK Science,* 8(1): 31-34

Nordstrom, M. L, Cnattingius, S. (1996). Effects on birthweights of maternal education, socioeconomic status, and work-related characteristics. *Scandinavian Journal of Social Medicine* 24:55-61

Mwabu, Germano (2008). "The Production of Child Health in Kenya: A Structural Model of Birth Weight." Yale *University Economic Growth Center Discussion Paper.* New Haven: Yale Economics Department Working Paper No. 52, 2008.

Okurut F. N. (2009). Determinants of Birth weight in Botswana. A Paper presented at the CSAE Conference, 22nd - 24th March 2009, University of Oxford, UK.

Parker, J. D., Schoendorf, K.C., Kiely, J. L. (1994). Associations between measures of socioeconomic status and low birth weight, small for gestational age, and premature delivery in the United States. *Annals of Epidemiology,* 4:271-278.

Phung H.,. Bauman, A. Nguyen, T. V, Young, L., Tran, M. and Hillman K. (2003). Risk Factors for Low Birth Weight in a Socio-Economically Disadvantaged Population: Parity, Marital Status, Ethnicity and Cigarette Smoking. *European Journal of Epidemiology,* 18(3):235-243

Rosenzweig, M. R., and Schultz, T.P (1982). The behavior of Mothers as Inputs to Child Health: The determinants of Birth Weight, Gestation, and the Rate of Fetal Growth, in Fuchs, V.R. (ed) *Economic Aspects of Health,* pp.53-92. Chicago: The University of Chicago Press.

Rosenzweig, M R., and Schultz, T. P (1983). Estimating a Household Production Function: Heterogeneity, the Demand for Health Inputs, and their Effects on Birth Weight. *Journal of Political Economy,* 91(5): 723 - 746.

Stephenson, T., Symonds, M. E. (2002). Maternal nutrition as a determinant of birth weight. *Arch Dis Child Fetal Neonatal Ed.* 86:F4-F6 doi:10.1136/fn.86.1.F4.

Ubomba-Jaswa, P and Ubomba-Jaswa, S. R. (1996). Correlates of low birth weight in Botswana. *South African Journal of Demography,* 6(1):64-73.

UNICEF, and WHO (2004). Low Birth Weight: Country, Regional and Global Estimates. New York: UNICEF.

UNICEF 2003 [http://www.unicef.org/spanish/pubsgen/sowc03/sowc03-sp.pdf, Accessed: June 5, 2011].

Vahdaninia, M., Tavafian, S. S. and Montazeri, A. (2008). Correlates of Low Birth Weight in Term Pregnancies: A retrospective Study from Iran. *BMC Pregnancy and Childbirth,* 8:12

Vogazianos, P; Fiala, J, Vogazianos, M. (2005). The Distribution of Birth Weights and their Determinants in the Republic of Cyprus for the period of 1990-2002", *Scripta Medica (BRNO),* 78(1): 31-44

Walton, A., Hammond, J. (1954). The maternal effects on growth and conformation in Shire horse-Sheltand pony crosses. *Proc R Soc Lond B Biol Sci,* 125:311–35.
WHO (2010). World Health Statistics 2010. World Health Organization, Geneva.
WHO (2011). World Health Statistics 2011. World Health Organization, Geneva.

2

Improving Newborn Interventions in Sub-Saharan Africa – Evaluating the Implementation Context in Uganda

Peter Waiswa

[1]*Makerere University School of Public Health, Department of Health Policy, Planning and Management,*
[2]*Department of Global Health, IHCAR, Division of Public Health, Karolinska Institutet*
[3]*Iganga/Mayuge Health and Demographic Surveillance Site*
[1,3]*Uganda*
[2]*Sweden*

1. Introduction

It has been proposed that the performance of a health system should be measured primarily by the effect on mortality. Childbirth is the time of greatest risk of mortality for a mother and a baby [1] and thus care at birth is a good marker of the performance of any health system. Yet every year, a staggering 7 million children die either in the first four weeks of life (3.8 million) or as still births (3.2 million) [2]. Despite this unbelievable magnitude of avoidable premature deaths, historically neonatal health was a forgotten area left in the cracks of safe motherhood and child health programs [1, 3-5].

The Millennium Development Goals (MDGs) that are directly related to newborn survival are MDGs 4 and 5. MDG 4 focuses on child survival and its target is to reduce under-5 child mortality by two-thirds by 2015, with a global target of 32 per 1000 live births [5, 6]. However, at current rates, most low income countries will not achieve this MDG target [6]. Available data shows that there has been no measurable reduction in early neonatal mortality in Sub-Saharan Africa (SSA) over the last decade, and the gap between the rich and the poor continues to widen [6]. Hence reducing neonatal deaths, especially early neonatal mortality is crucial to meeting MDG 4 [1]. However, evidence shows that most of the neonatal deaths are intimately linked to maternal problems especially those related to the management of the intra-partum period [1, 7, 8]. A solution addressing both maternal and newborn health is cost-effective.

Although we have an estimate of the huge magnitude of neonatal deaths and their importance to achieve MDG 4 target in the next few years to 2015, SSA has had no measurable reduction in neonatal deaths for about a decade now [5, 6]. This despite the existence of evidence that low cost interventions that have the potential to reduce neonatal mortality by 41–72% worldwide [8]; and most of these are relatively simple [9].

In order to accelerate efforts towards achieving MDG 4, a number of SSA countries including Uganda are designing programs to integrate newborn interventions into current maternal and newborn programs, hitherto a neglected area. Most of these efforts are based on global recommendations. Moreover, most of the evidence is based on small scale studies from Asia and a few from South America, and none to date from SSA. In fact, WHO and UNICEF have already recommended community based interventions through home visits as one of the key strategies [10]. Yet it is known that the health system context including cultures and practices in SSA is different from that in Asia. However, we know that there is no magic "one size fits all" program to address neonatal mortality. Many countries such as Uganda have already translated this evidence into policy. However, evidence or policy on paper does not usually translate into practice, leading to the so called "know-do-gap" or the "knowledge-implementation gap" [11]. The local epidemiology as well as health system design and performance and community demand are key factors that need to be considered [12, 13]. This is crucial for identifying and recognizing the extent of the "know-do-gap" in current programs.

Key "knowledge-implementation gaps" related to neonatal health at the implementation level in SSA health systems include: identifying missed opportunities or modifiable delays within the health care delivery system that lead to newborn deaths; understanding whether the evidence-based globally recommended practices are acceptable in the local context (home care practices, community perceptions and underlying cultural beliefs); and the current uptake of neonatal interventions including the quality of newborn care gaps across the maternal and newborn care continuum.

In this paper, I assess the implementation context for evidence-based newborn interventions, namely, primary health care health facilities, households/communities, and the linkages there of in the continuum for maternal and newborn care in terms of time and place), in order to inform program design and policy. The findings described in the paper were used to design the Uganda Newborn trial (UNEST) (trial register ICRCTN 50321130)

2. Methods

2.1 Study area and population

The studies described here were conducted in Iganga and Mayuge districts (Figure 1), which are part of the Busoga region, and situated in the south-eastern part of Uganda. Including Iganga and Mayuge, the Busoga region has seven administrative districts – the others being Bugiri, Kamuli, Kaliro, Namutumba and Jinja. Busoga region is composed of 11 principalities of the Basoga tribe and is one of the largest traditional kingdoms of Uganda. Study II, III, and the health facility component of IV, where conducted in the Iganga/Mayuge health and demographic surveillance system (HDSS), whereas study I, and the qualitative component of study IV, were conducted elsewhere outside the surveillance area in the two districts of Iganga and Mayuge. Busoga region has a population of about 2.8 million people, of mixed tribal identification, and represents approximately 8.4% of the Ugandan population, living in an area of about 7100 sq. miles. To the west of the Basoga tribe live the Baganda tribe, the largest tribe of Uganda. However, their two languages, traditional practices and cultures are similar to each other.

Iganga/Mayuge HDSS is situated in the Eastern part of Uganda, and it covers an area across the two districts of Iganga and Mayuge. This area covers 155sqkm, comprising 18 parishes and 65 villages. At the time of data collection, the Health Demographic Surveillance System

(HDSS) population was about 68,000 people, staying in roughly 12,000 households. The average household size is five persons per household, and the main occupation is subsistence agriculture.

The HDSS is comprised largely of a rural area with only Iganga town council being peri-urban. The HDSS is currently expanding to new areas along with an increase in the specific demands for more research.

In Iganga/Mayuge HDSS, there is one general hospital, 15 health centres, about two dozen small private clinics and other informal health providers, mostly traditional birth attendants, drug shops and private clinics that are most often found in small trading centres, as well as in Iganga proper (Figure 5). All government and NGO facilities have clinical officers and nurses for health care delivery, apart from delivery provided by the hospital, which also has doctors. Malaria is endemic, and pneumonia is prevalent in the district.

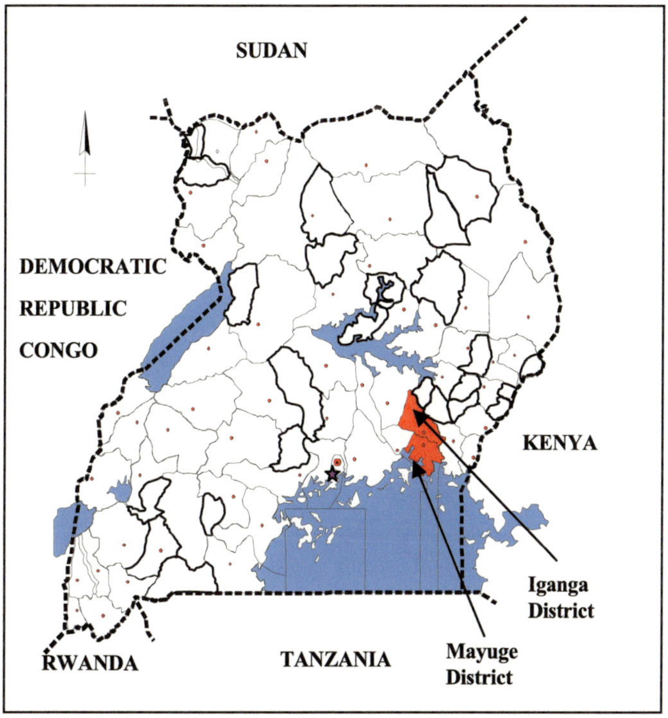

Fig. 1. Map of Uganda showing the location of Iganga and Mayuge Districts

2.2 Study design, sampling and data collection

This paper summarises four studies, with a general aim to inform design of a newborn intervention as tailored to the local context. This was a cross-sectional study with both qualitative and quantitative methods of analysis. The studies were designed such that they complement one another. An assessment was done of causes of newborn deaths, and identified where major delays occurred as they contribute to death. Exploration of the acceptability of the evidence-based newborn practices, and it helped to inform the design of the variables that assessed uptake of newborn care practices among babies who survived the neonatal period. Finally, the picture was completed by seeking to understand the care provided to preterm babies at home and in health facilities as an example of the current care for newborn babies in the study area. Table 1 summarises the studies, their designs and sample sizes.

Study objective	Methods	Study population and sample size
Acceptability of evidence-based newborn care practices	10 FGDs and 10 KI interviews	Mothers, fathers, grandparents Child minders Total 98 people
Uptake of newborn care practices	Cross-sectional population based study	Mothers of babies 1-4 months N=414
Modifiable delays leading to newborn deaths	Case series	Neonatal deaths N=64
Care of preterm babies	Health facility survey IDIs FGDs	1 hospital and 15 health units 11 CHWs 10 mothers of preterm babies 6 fathers of preterm babies 3 grandmothers of preterm babies 3 FGDs

Table 1. Summary of methods

2.3 Qualitative studies

2.3.1 Acceptability of evidence-based newborn care practices

A qualitative approach was used to explore the aacceptability of evidence-based neonatal care practices in rural Uganda. Ten FGDs were conducted as follows: two with younger mothers less than 30 years; four with older mothers more than 30 years or having grandchildren; two with fathers and another two with child minders (older children who take care of other children) of up to 13 years of age. Selection of young mothers and fathers was limited to those having children less than six months of age in order to ensure that responses reflect recent/current practices. In addition, we also conducted key-informant interviews (KIs) with six health workers and four traditional birth attendants (TBAs). Villages were selected for interviews from both near and far from the hospital to represent the rural-urban divide. Using guidelines from the research team, community leaders identified participants for the FGDs, and district leaders of health services identified health workers and TBAs for the KIs. Pre-tested checklists guided discussions about the acceptability and barriers to adapting practices within the continuum of care approach [14-16] with special focus on ANC, intra-partum care, and postnatal care for the mother and the baby, and to home visits by a volunteer to promote improved care during pregnancy, delivery and in the postnatal period. Participants were asked to present their own experiences and actions, or otherwise to describe general attitudes.

2.3.2 Care of preterm babies

In order to understand the perceptions and care of preterm babies at home and at health facilities, three different methods were used in order to triangulate findings: participant observations [17], focus-group discussions and in-depth interviews (IDIs). Field work took place in two sub-counties in each district. The respondents for each method are shown in table 2.

Method of data collection	Number of subjects/interviews/groups
Health facility observations	16 health facilities
In-depth interviews	n = 31
Community health workers (CHWs)	8
Traditional birth attendants (TBAs)	4
Mothers of preterm babies	10
Fathers of preterm babies	6
Grandmothers of preterm babies	3
Focus group discussions	
Health workers	1 FGD (six midwives/nurses)
Men	1 FGD (8 men)
Women	1 FGD (10 women)

Table 2. Respondents/subjects and methods

A neonatal midwife from a tertiary hospital worked in health units for a month while also observing health workers, care givers and events to find out about behaviours and interactions using a semi-structured checklist and also recorded both peculiar and mundane activities and observations in a field diary [17].

IDIs were conducted with 8 CHWs (3 community drug distributors, 2 breastfeeding peer educators, and 4 safe motherhood volunteers). Ten preterm babies originating from the study areas were identified from among 42 preterm births recorded in the hospital over a six months period and traced at home for interviews. Three mothers could not be traced. Three mothers of preterm birth which occurred at home where identified by community members for interview. We conducted interviews till we realized saturation- that is we continued interviews till no new information came up. We also interviewed 6 fathers and 3 grandmothers. Finally, we conducted 3 FGDs one for midwives in the hospital and two in the community with parents but not necessarily of preterm babies (one FGD for men and one for women) to get general community perceptions. Towards the end of each community FGD, participants were shown pictures of a mother practicing kangaroo mother care (KMC) in order to assess knowledge, perceptions and acceptability.

2.4 Quantitative studies

2.4.1 Uptake of newborn care practices

A population-based cross-sectional was conducted among women with a baby aged 1-4 months (n=414) in order to determine socioeconomic differences in uptake of newborn care practices. Socio-demographic and household socio-economic status (SES) information were collected in a separate survey a year earlier. The tool was pre-tested among 25 mothers attending a postnatal clinic at the local hospital. Mothers who had had a stillbirth or a neonatal death were not interviewed for this study.

2.4.2 Modifiable delays leading to newborn deaths

For all deaths occurring in the DSS, community informants, locally known as community scouts, report to interviewers. After a period of 4-6 weeks of mourning, a verbal and social autopsy questionnaire was administered by one of three trained native interviewers to a close caregiver of the deceased. Sixty-four newborn deaths were investigated covering the period January 2005-December 2008. In addition, a health facility survey was conducted in all 16 major public and private health facilities serving the DSS, which included a general hospital. Data were collected on physical infrastructure, staff inventory, and on the presence of essential and desirable equipment for newborn care. Finally, knowledge assessment on maternal and newborn care was conducted using a self-administered questionnaire adapted from one used for a similar study [18]. The assessment was conducted among 52 health providers selected proportionally to represent level of care.

Two experienced, practicing physicians independently reviewed each death and assigned cause of death using a hierarchical approach [19]. Whenever there was a disagreement, they met to review the case, and if agreement was reached, the diagnosis was accepted as the definitive cause of death. However, if this was not possible, the cause of death was coded as undetermined. We defined delays as follows: Delay 1, which is the delay to recognise illness and the need to seek medical care, included any newborn baby who died at home or where it took more than 12 hours to seek outside care; Delay 2, the transport delay, included newborn babies whose care givers expressed problems with getting transport; and Delay 3, the delay in receiving quality care, included delay in receiving or failure to receive quality care at a health facility (as judged by the audit physician).

2.5 Data analysis

For the qualitative studies, analysis of the in-depth interviews, key informant interviews and FGDs used latent thematic content analysis. Transcripts were first read several times to get an overall picture and then meaningful units were coded, condensed and categorized into broad themes [20]. Barriers to care seeking were characterized according to the three delays model which includes delays in deciding to seek care, delay in reaching the health facility, and delay in receiving care once at the health facility [21, 22]. Relevant quotes were extracted and some were presented verbatim.

For the quantitative data, univariate, bavariate and multi-variate analysis with logistic regression was done in stata 10. Households were stratified into quintiles of socioeconomic status. Data on newborn care practices was analysed through creating the following composite outcomes: good neonatal feeding, good cord care, and optimal thermal care. This was done by combining related individual practices from a list of twelve antenatal/essential newborn care practices. Multiple logistic regression analysis was used to identify determinants of each dichotomised composite outcome.

Ethical approval for all studies was given by the Uganda National Council for Science and Technology following review by the Institutional Review Board of Makerere University School of Public Health. Verbal autopsy is culturally sensitive, interviews are conducted 4-6 weeks after a death occurred in order to allow a period of mourning as per local customs. Interviewers were recruited locally and trained to respect cultural issues. In all the four studies, all moderators and interviewers were experienced and their minimum education was to diploma level for moderators and twelve years of formal education for interviewers. Verbal informed consent was sought and obtained from all participants.

3. Results

3.1 Similar low uptake of essential newborn care practices among the poorest and least poor

In general, there were low levels of coverage of the desired practices (table 3). A total of 46% of the respondents delivered in the hospital or in a health unit, 26% delivered in private clinics (most informal with unqualified staff and poor infrastructure) and 28% at home or with a TBA. Cord cutting was done mostly by use of a razorblade (67%) of which 11% were reused, and only 28% reported to have used cord scissors. About half of the mothers put substances on the cord (such as powder, surgical spirit, salty water, or lizard droppings). To keep warm, 86% babies were immediately wrapped, but skin-to-skin (STS) care was almost non-existent (2%). Early bathing was the norm, with 56% of the babies bathed within the first 6 hours, 82% within the first 12 hours, and almost all during the first 24 hours. Although all babies were breastfed, only about half were initiated within the first hour of birth, with 41% initiating within 1 - 6 hours. Other feeds besides breast milk including cow's milk, plain water, sugar or glucose water, gripe water and tea were given to 35% of babies in the neonatal period, contrary to recommendations.

Table 4 shows the independent predictors of safe cord care. Multiparous mothers were less likely to have good cord practices when compared to primiparas (OR 0.5, CI 0.3 - 0.9); and so were mothers whose labour began at night compared to those whose labour began during day time (OR 0.6, CI 0.4 - 0.9). Although significantly more mothers in the high SES delivered in health facilities (p < 000), we found that place of delivery did not predict any of the ENC practices assessed.

Characteristics	Total	%
Time labour began n= 356		
Day	146	42
Night	205	58
Time of delivery n=391		
Day	195	50
Night	196	50
Health facility delivery n=393		
Yes	181	46
No	212	54
Surface of delivery n=392		
Clean	258	66
Dirty	134	34
Instrument used to cut the cord n=391		
Clean	333	85
Not clean	58	15
Material used to tie the cord n=391		
Clean	387	99
Not clean	4	1

Characteristics	Total	%
Type of instrument used to cut the cord n=391		
Un used new razor blade	223	57
Used razor blade	41	10
Scissors	110	28
Other/ Don't know	17	5.0
What was used to tie the cord n=391		
Cloth strip	39	10.0
Clean thread	338	86.4
Rubber band	3	0.1
Other/Don't know	11	2.8
What was put on the cord n=389		
Nothing	198	51
Medical drugs	11	3.0
Powder	87	22.2
Ash	3	0.8
Salty water	43	11
Other	47	12
How long after birth baby was breastfed n=392		
Immediately	199	51
Less than 6 hours	159	41
6 – 24 hours	24	6.0
>24 hours	10	2.0
If at all, bottle fed in neonatal period n=391		
Yes	42	11
No	349	89
How long after birth was baby first bathed n=244		
Less than 1 hour	13	5
2- 6 hours	125	51
7 - 12 hours	63	26
13 - 24 hours	34	14
>24 hours	9	4
Safe cord care n=387		
Yes	149	39
No	238	61
Good neonatal feeding n=378		
Yes	216	57
No	162	43
Optimal thermal care n=398		
Yes	166	42
No	226	58

Table 3. Level of selected care practices during delivery and neonatal period

Variable	Univariate Unadjusted		Multivariate Adjusted*	
	OR	95% CI	OR	95% CI
Maternal Age				
<19	1		1	
19-25	0.52	0.24-1.11	0.68	0.31-1.51
26-30	0.47	0.21-1.03	0.62	0.26-1.47
>30	0.89	0.41-1.93	1.19	0.48-2.95
Parity				
1	1			
2-4	0.44	0.25-0.76	0.45	0.25-0.79
>4	0.68	0.40-1.13	0.57	0.30-1.08
Time labour began				
Day	1			
Night	0.66	0.44-1.01	0.61	0.0 -0.94

*Adjusted for maternal age, parity and time labour began
* p for the whole model = 0.003

Table 4. Logistic models with safe cord care practices as dependent variable versus all independent variables having significant chi-square values in bivariate analysis

3.2 Newborn babies die close to time of birth due to care-seeking delays

Of the 64 newborn deaths investigated, 37% (24/64) had been born in a hospital or a health centre, 23% (15/64) in a private clinic and 39% (25/64) at a TBA, at home or on the way to hospital. Of these deaths, 47% (30/64) occurred within the first 24 hours after birth and 78% in the first week, and only 22% occurred in the remaining three weeks of the neonatal period (Figure 6). The median age at death was two days (IQR 1-4). During the same period, most births were reportedly conducted by a trained health worker (58%, 37/64). Twenty deaths (33%) occurred either in a hospital or a health centre, 8 (13%) in a clinic, with the majority (54%) dying away from a health facility (TBA, at home or on the way to hospital).

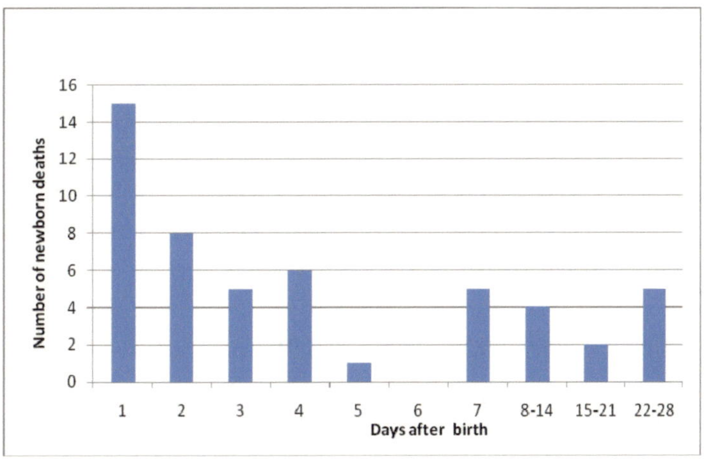

Fig. 2. Distribution of newborn deaths by day after birth in Iganga/Mayuge DSS, eastern Uganda

The leading causes of death were sepsis or pneumonia (31%), birth asphyxia (30%) and preterm birth (25%) (Figure 3). Delay in problem recognition/deciding to seek care outside the home (Delay 1) was the greatest contributor to deaths (50%, 32/64). Most newborn babies who died had started being unwell during or immediately after birth (57%, 36/64), and were unwell for a short period, with the median duration of illness being two days (IQR 1-6). Care-seeking was generally delayed, with the median duration to seeking care from outside the home being three days from illness onset (IQR 1-6 days).

The second major contributor to newborn deaths was delay in receiving quality care at the health facility (Delay 3) (30%, 19/64). A total of 53% (9/17) newborns that were taken outside the home for care reportedly made contact with a qualified health worker, but five caretakers went to drug shops and one to a spiritual leader.

Surprisingly, the transport delay to a health facility (Delay 2) was found to be a main contributor to only 20% (13/64) of newborn deaths. A second delay was identified as being a contributor to 22% of the newborn deaths investigated.

The major causes of death by main contributing delay were as follows: Delay 1 - sepsis or pneumonia (32%) followed by birth asphyxia (22%); Delay 2 - birth asphyxia (46%) followed by sepsis or pneumonia (31%); Delay 3 - preterm births (37%) followed by birth asphyxia (32%).

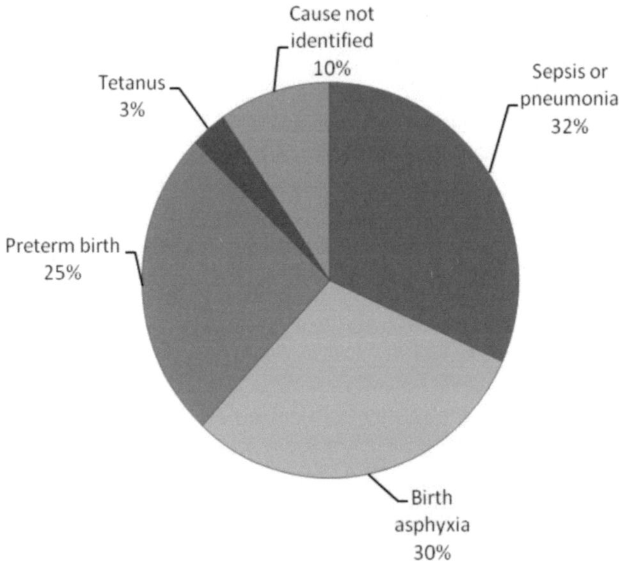

Fig. 3. Primary causes of newborn deaths

3.3 Readiness of health facilities for newborn care

Health facilities had just about half of the minimum Ministry of Health recommended qualified health workers, and almost all lacked the basic newborn equipment, drugs, supplies and an effective referral system. For instance, only 44% (7/16) of health facilities had a delivery kit, 44% (7/16) had a neonatal weighing scale, and only 6% (1/16) had a neonatal resuscitation kit.

Overall, in the knowledge assessment, participants were correct for only 58% of the questions across the maternal and newborn care continuum. Medical assistants/clinical officers had the best mean score (63%), followed by registered midwives (61%), enrolled midwives (56.5%) and enrolled nurses (50%). Participants were correct mostly for questions on ANC (65%), followed by intra-partum care (52%); the least correct answers were on newborn/postnatal care (31%).

These poor newborn care practices were confirmed in the qualitative studies. Findings from interviews revealed that most evidence-based newborn care practices were acceptable to community members; however exceptions do exist especially around dry cord care and delayed bathing. Most preterm babies are cared for at home, however, care practices are not only inadequate but also potentially harmful. A number of mothers are using powder and antiseptics for the cord, sugar or glucose water for initiation of feeding and bottles to feed babies. Health facilities lacked capacity (in terms of skilled staff, equipment, drugs, protocols and supplies) for newborn care.

4. Discussion

These studies explored both preventive and curative care for all newborn babies, at home and in health facilities, as well as related care-seeking delays contributing to newborn deaths in two districts of Uganda. Most evidence-based newborn care practices were acceptable to community members, however exceptions do exist. Newborn care practices were of poor quality and coverage was low across all socio-economic groups. Delays in problem recognition and decision-making (Delay 1), together with poor quality care at health facilities (Delay 3) were found to be the major delays related to newborn death in this setting. Most preterm babies are cared for at home, however, care practices are not only inadequate but also potentially harmful. A number of mothers are using powder and antiseptics for the cord, sugar or glucose water for initiation of feeding and bottles to feed babies. Health facilities lack capacity (in terms of skilled staff, equipment, drugs, protocols and supplies) for newborn care. These findings have important policy and programmatic implications for informing the design and delivery of evidence-based newborn interventions in Uganda, and other similar settings.

4.1 Poor coverage and quality of newborn care practices

The overall level of coverage of newborn care practices was low when assessed as composite outcomes Of newborns, 46% had a facility delivery, and when assessed as composite outcomes only 38% were judged to have had good cord care, 42% had optimal thermal care, and only 57% were considered to have had adequate neonatal feeding. The low coverage levels of composite outcomes were contrary to that of some individual practices. For instance, good cord care as a composite outcome had a coverage of only 38%, and yet use of a clean instrument to cut the umbilical cord (85%) and clean thread to tie the cord (90%) were high, but no substance applied to the cord was low (51%). The trend was similar for optimal breastfeeding and good thermal care. Thus, coverage of some practices might be high when assessed as individual practices, but quite low when evaluated as composite practices. These findings imply that, put together, i.e. assessed as composite outcomes, the majority of newborn babies are not accessing adequate preventive practices.

The coverage of adequate newborn care practices was not influenced by place of delivery. These findings differ from those reported from rural Uttar Pradesh [23], where it was found that ANC and skilled attendance were associated with clean cord care and early breastfeeding.

The findings indicate that although almost all mothers breastfed their babies, about half of the infants were not breastfed within the first one hour as is recommended [24], thereby putting these neonates at an increased risk for death [25]. In addition, more than one-third of respondents reported that they gave feeds other than breast milk in the neonatal period. A study by Engebretsen et al. conducted in eastern Uganda [26] found that only 7% of infants were exclusively breastfed by age three months. In other words, both their study and ours show that as early as the neonatal period, over one-third of infants are not exclusively breastfed. The low coverage of essential newborn care practices means that the prevent aspect of care for the newborn is weak, and needs strengthening.

The coverage of composite newborn care practices did not differ between the least poor and the poorest, i.e. coverage seemed not to be modified by socioeconomic status. This was despite good physical access to health facilities. Usually, mortality is higher and coverage is lower among the poorest [27]. Further, it has been documented elsewhere that universal interventions often reach the least poor first and the poorest later [28], but this was not the case here.

There are several possible explanations for the lack of differences in coverage across socioeconomic groupings. First, in the study setting, there were no specific programmes promoting newborn care in the study districts during the previous five years (and therefore even the least poor were not accessing the desired care practices). Secondly, it may be that SES classifications in quintiles as based on assets (such as type of material used for floors in houses or as possession such as a bicycle) may not classify people in relation to newborn care practices. The study lacked power to find a difference in composite newborn care practices by SES.

4.2 Acceptability of evidence-based newborn care practices at community level

Despite the low coverage of newborn care practices shown above, most of the globally recommended newborn care practices were acceptable to community members (mothers, fathers, grandmothers, grandfathers and CHWs), but they were not well promoted by providers which might be the explanation for the low coverage. On the other hand, the majority of women reported that they would prefer to have a health facility delivery, although in practice women often did not manage, mainly because of a number of barriers, including costs, distances, rude health workers and the challenges of accessing health care at night. These same challenges were identified in two recent published reviews as contributing to care-seeking delays for delivery care [29, 30].

Among the globally recommended evidence-based newborn care practices, a few were deemed to be less acceptable to most community members. For example, although the WHO guidelines recommend that nothing should be put on the cord [31], and that bathing of babies should be delayed, this was not deemed acceptable many community members or health care providers because of various perceptions or barriers. The perceived need for early bathing was of the newborn is strong in this community. Some of the reasons given included a belief that putting substances on the cord helps the cord to "heal fast", and that "babies are born dirty" or that mothers expected "visitors to find the baby clean". A study in Tanzania showed that many communities support the notion that the umbilical cord is thought to make the baby vulnerable to witchcraft, and great care is therefore taken to shield both the mother and baby from bad spirits until the cord falls off. Such forms of 'protection' include applying drugs, cow dung, and powder to help heal the cord. Bathing also plays a role here, and babies are bathed early, sometimes with cold water [32]. Studies in South Asia have reported similar findings, including unhygienic cord cutting and care, as well as early bathing [23, 33-36]. The implication of these findings is that interventions to promote dry cord care and delayed bathing must focus on both the individual and the community.

The finding that some globally recommended evidence-based newborn care practices might not be acceptable, and are therefore not promoted or implemented at the community level, raises the issue of "fit" and whether or not "evidence-based" interventions actually fit in the local implementation context (referred to as 'glocal'). There is no "one size fits all" to neonatal survival [12], and interventions proved effective in one setting, may, in another setting, need to be preceded by local adaptation so as to be 'tailored' to the local context before being scaled up [4, 37, 38]. This is important for understanding the "black box of implementation" [39, 40] A compromise of practices might be needed, such as wiping instead of early bathing, or applying a safe substance to the umbilical cord (such as chlorhexidine) [41, 42].

4.3 Delays contributing to newborn deaths

As pathological causes, sepsis or pneumonia, followed by birth asphyxia, and then preterm births were the leading causes of death overall, as reported elsewhere for low income countries [5, 43]. However, as 'social causes' of deaths, when the modified three delays model [22]was applied, the findings showed that 50% of newborn deaths were mainly related to recognise delay (Delay 1 or delay in illness recognition and deciding to seek outside care), and 30% were due to treat (Delay 3 or poor quality care at health facilities), while 20% were due to access or transport problems (Delay 2). The delay to seek seemed not to be a major problem in the study setting due to a relatively good physical access to health facilities, which may not be the same across Uganda. Together, delays recognise and treat contributed to 80% of the newborn babies who died. These findings on the contribution of delays to newborn death differ from those in a Tanzanian study by Mbaruku and colleagues, which was one of the first studies to apply the three delays model to perinatal death [44]. The latter reported that most newborns died as a result of the third delay; however, Mbaruku's study only collected data from the hospital and did not include older neonates (>1 week).

4.3.1 Delay 1: Delays in problem recognition and delays in deciding to seek care

Of the newborn babies who did not die on the day of birth, most deaths occurred following delays at home. The majority were sick for at least three days before care was sought outside the home. Nearly half of the at-home deaths resulted from sepsis or pneumonia (III). According to the original model by Thaddeus and Maine [22], delays at home could be a reflection of problem recognition or a delay in deciding to seek care. Given the fact that newborn babies are very vulnerable, a delay of three days which we found before seeking care outside the home is grave, and such sick newborns may not be helped by weak health facilities.

A recent ethnographic study in Ghana found that mothers might not be able to recognise serious illness in their newborns, and they also often do not seek care outside the home even when they do recognise serious illness [45]. It seems that even when parents are made to recognise the need to seek outside care, decision-making can be problematic. An intervention trial in Bangladesh, in which CHWs conducted intense surveillance of sick newborns, identified two challenges especially for young neonates: reaching neonates within the first two days after birth and 'parental compliance with advice to seek outside care' [46]. Studies in older children conducted in the same setting [47, 48], and elsewhere in Uganda [49], have identified challenges to care-seeking as mainly related to cost.

From the above it is clear that efforts to improve newborn survival in Uganda must address 'Delay 1' delays related to recognition and decision-making.

4.3.2 Delay 2: Delay in reaching a health facility

Of newborn babies who died, 20% were related to Delay 2, and the main cause of death was birth asphyxia . The seemingly low contribution of transport delays to babies who died may be explained by the fact that the study setting had generally good physical access to health services, and availability of bicycles and motorcycles as means of referral was good. However, for transportation to be effective, it must also be of the right quality. A limitation of the second delay as originally presented by Thaddeus and Maine [22] is that it does not call for assessing the quality of transportation. Transport of seriously ill children has been identified as an important but neglected issue in global health [50]. There is evidence that morbidity and mortality of critically ill patients are much reduced if specially trained teams availed transport and delivered life-saving treatments [51, 52]. However, such transport facilities cannot be met by the current bicycle and motorcycle services in the area. As such, transport for seriously sick children needs to be improved.

4.3.3 Delay 3: Delay in receiving quality care at a health facility

In total, 33% of newborn deaths were attributed to health facility-related delays and resulted mainly from prematurity (37%), followed by birth asphyxia (32%). The health facility assessment conducted in the area showed inadequacy in the number of qualified providers. Further, available providers lacked knowledge about managing newborn babies. A knowledge assessment on care during pregnancy, delivery and postnatal care showed the average score to be low, especially on questions related to newborn care (31%). These findings are similar to those reported elsewhere in low income countries [18, 53]. The health facility assessment also showed a general lack of basic newborn equipment, drugs (injectable ampicillin and gentamycin), supplies and an effective referral system. For instance, only 44% (7/16) of health facilities had a delivery kit, 44% (7/16) had a neonatal weighing scale and only 6% (1/16) had a neonatal resuscitation kit. Thirteen percent of newborn deaths occurred in small private clinics; where capacity to manage the newborn was also very weak. Similarly, a recent study of Kenyan hospitals also found that these did not have a capacity to manage sick newborn babies [54].

Thus, in terms of the three delays model, a lack of skilled staff, protocols, drugs and equipment coupled with weak management often lead to treat delays in providing quality care for sick babies as well as other newborns at risk of death, such as those with birth asphyxia or prematurity. The risk of deaths for newborn babies is made even worse when one considers that in Uganda, it is currently presumed that sick newborn babies can only be managed at higher level health facilities. This effectively means that because of policy regulations, the lowest level of health facilities (HC-IIs) are not allowed to have the basic newborn drugs and equipment, and their role in care is thereby limited to the initiation of treatment prior to referral. Such limitations remain, despite the fact that well documented, evidence-based constraints to care-seeking for sick children to attend health facilities have been identified [47, 48, 55-61]. Thus, reducing the treat delay by bringing qualified staff, equipment, antibiotics, supplies and guidelines to improve newborn care at health facilities of all levels is critical for newborn survival in this setting.

4.4 Addressing the delays that lead to newborn deaths

The findings suggest that besides problem recognition, referral for sick newborns also needs to be improved, both from the community and from first level health facilities, as findings show that most caretakers of sick newborns do not comply with referral advice. To improve newborn survival, interventions need to address both supply and demand-side practices and care. Thus, there is a need to strengthen both health facility and community programmes if newborn care is to be improved in low-income countries [8, 15, 62, 63]. To reduce newborn death, addressing delay 1 or delay in problem recognition and in deciding to seek outside care will be critical, as it was a major contributor to half of the deaths investigated in this study.

Based on a number of small efficacy studies, almost all from Asia [62, 64-66], efforts to scale up newborn care in low income countries through community based interventions are gathering pace. Community-based interventions can address delays in problem recognition of sick newborns (delay 1) by promoting supervised deliveries, birth preparedness and raising awareness on maternal and newborn danger signs. These are some of the practices we have found to be deficient in this setting [67]. However, unless community interventions include treatment and care at home, their success will mainly depend on strengthening of health facilities so that women in labour and sick newborn babies receive quality care. It has been suggested that introducing maternal and perinatal audit in health facilities [68], and improving neonatal resuscitation skills among health workers [69] are effective strategies to address quality of care issues for newborn babies. However, operationalising this in low-income countries remains a challenge as recent reviews have shown that the understanding of how to reduce health facility based newborn deaths is still limited [70, 71].

4.5 Perceptions and care for preterm and other newborn babies

The study on preterm care demonstrated several missed opportunities for health promotion activities to improve care of preterm and other low birth weight babies. Mothers were doing their best to care for preterm babies, but care practices were of poor quality and potentially harmful. At community level and in health facilities, including the general hospital, no STS or KMC was practiced. To keep warm, e.g. babies were wrapped in many clothes. Although most preterm babies were managed at home, care practices were of poor quality. For instance, and in addition to practices already mentioned, mothers reported using hot objects such as jerry cans filled with hot water and charcoal stoves to keep preterm babies warm. Therefore, these mothers perceived preterm babies as needing special care.

Furthermore, information from interviews showed that community members were generally not fatalistic in their attitudes, as was also found in Malawi [72]. Thus, in terms of the TRA, the mothers had a positive attitude towards preterm care, meaning that if health providers took advantage of this opportunity to promote newborn care practices, the chances of them being accepted was likely to be high (high outcome expectancy). However, missing was the promotion of desired practices by caregivers. Recent reviews have re-emphasised the importance of implementing interventions to improve the care of preterm births, which is not only the leading direct cause of neonatal mortality, but also accounts for an estimated 27% neonatal deaths every year and is a risk factor for many neonatal deaths resulting from other causes such as infections [43]. Providers of health care should take advantage of this perceived positive attitude towards preterm babies by promoting the recommended care practices at both health facility and community levels.

A number of mothers were putting powder or antiseptics, among other substances, on the cord, and were using a bottle to feed the baby or were mixing/replacing breastfeeding (especially at initiation of feeding) with various substitutes such as glucose or sugar water or honey. Whether these are replacing other "more dangerous" practices, such as putting cow dung, dust or ash on the cord (as prevalent in the study area in the past) could not be shown in a cross-sectional study. But powder, antiseptics and bottle feeding are relatively new phenomena.

Similar 'new' practices have also been reported from Bangladesh [34], India [33] and Tanzania [32]. Moran and colleagues reported that women apply several substances to the cord including talcum powder and savlon (an antiseptic liquid). In addition, initiation of breastfeeding is often done by giving other substances such as honey and sugar water, and the authors suggest that such practices are a consequence of increasing urbanisation [34]. The Uganda Demographic Health Survey [73] and a study from western Uganda found that use of pre-lacteals was common even among educated mothers [74]. Studies on breastfeeding patterns in low income countries suggest that changes in breastfeeding have been influenced by marketing of formula milk, urbanisation, and the need for women to work away from home [75]. Thus, applying the TRA, these findings seem to suggest that within a changing environment the practices of mothers may be influenced by perceived social norms in which caregivers are aware of the expected behaviour and are willing to comply with such expectations, that is, they may associate some of these practices with 'modernity'. If these assumptions are true, then the implication is for a need for interventions targeting the entire population so as to diffuse the perceived social norms that are evolving. Here, the example of infant formula replacing breastfeeding is a warning example of how 'modern' practice with commercial interests can lead to a practice transition [76, 77].

5. Conclusion

Newborn care practices are generally poor across all socio-economic groups. This is despite the fact that most evidence-based newborn care practices were acceptable to community members although a few were not deemed acceptable. Delays occur at all levels of the continuum of care including home, access and at health facilities. The design of interventions for the implementation of evidence-based newborn care practices needs to be tailored to the local context. In order to reduce newborn deaths, a universal strategy targeting the entire population is needed and should utilise the many missed opportunities in current programmes. Capacity to manage newborns should be built at health facilities, including private clinics and those at the lower level. Community health workers in health facility-linked preventive and curative newborn programmes may assist in underserved areasPolicymakers need to mitigate a possible newborn care practices transition in which "suboptimal" practices are being replaced with "modern" practices. This can be done through proper training, provision of clear guidelines and support for health workers, and by especially ensuring that health facilities have adequate supplies.

Implementation research on how to reduce care-seeking delays and improve referral and care at home and in both private and public health facilities for newborn babies is recommended. In addition, exploration should be done on how to best integrate CHWs into maternal and newborn care in health facility-linked programs, especially the interface with primary level health facilities. Such an intervention, the Uganda Newborn trial (UNEST) (trial register ICRCTN 50321130), was designed based on the findings described in this paper and implemented in the two study districts. The study is thus an example of research-to-programmes and policy, since results and experiences from each stage are constantly fed to policy makers.

6. References

[1] Lawn, J.E., et al., *Two million intrapartum-related stillbirths and neonatal deaths: Where, why, and what can be done?* Int J Gynaecol Obstet, 2009.

[2] Unicef, *State of the World's Children 2009*2009, New York: UNICEF.

[3] Bhutta, Z.A., *Beyond Bellagio: addressing the challenge of sustainable child health in developing countries.* Arch Dis Child, 2004. 89(5): p. 483-7.

[4] Bhutta, Z.A., et al., *Alma-Ata: Rebirth and Revision 6 Interventions to address maternal, newborn, and child survival: what difference can integrated primary health care strategies make?* Lancet, 2008. 372(9642): p. 972-89.

[5] Lawn, J.E., S. Cousens, and J. Zupan, *4 million neonatal deaths: when? Where? Why?* Lancet, 2005. 365(9462): p. 891-900.

[6] Bryce, J., et al., *Countdown to 2015 for maternal, newborn, and child survival: the 2008 report on tracking coverage of interventions.* Lancet, 2008. 371(9620): p. 1247-58.

[7] Harvey, S.A., et al., *Pharmacological approaches to defining the role of chaperones in aging and prostate cancer progression.* Cell Stress Chaperones, 2002. 7(2): p. 230-4.

[8] Darmstadt, G.L., et al., *Evidence-based, cost-effective interventions: how many newborn babies can we save?* Lancet, 2005. 365(9463): p. 977-88.

[9] Adam, T., et al., *Cost effectiveness analysis of strategies for maternal and neonatal health in developing countries.* BMJ, 2005. 331(7525): p. 1107.

[10] World Health Organization. Dept. of Child and Adolescent Health and Development. and UNICEF., *Home visits for the newborn child : a strategy to improve survival : WHO/UNICEF joint statement*2009, Geneva: World Health Organization. 7 p.

[11] Sanders, D. and A. Haines, *Implementation research is needed to achieve international health goals.* PLoS Med, 2006. 3(6): p. e186.

[12] Knippenberg, R., et al., *Systematic scaling up of neonatal care in countries.* Lancet, 2005. 365(9464): p. 1087-98.

[13] Travis, P., et al., *Overcoming health-systems constraints to achieve the Millennium Development Goals.* Lancet, 2004. 364(9437): p. 900-6.
[14] Marsh, D.R., et al., *Advancing newborn health and survival in developing countries: a conceptual framework.* J Perinatol, 2002. 22(7): p. 572-6.
[15] Kerber, K.J., et al., *Continuum of care for maternal, newborn, and child health: from slogan to service delivery.* Lancet, 2007. 370(9595): p. 1358-69.
[16] Tinker, A., et al., A continuum of care to save newborn lives. Lancet, 2005. 365(9462): p. 822-5.
[17] Mays N, P.C., *Qualitative Research: Observational methods in health care settings.* British Medical Journal, 1995. 311: p. 182-184.
[18] Harvey, S.A., et al., *Are skilled birth attendants really skilled? A measurement method, some disturbing results and a potential way forward.* Bull World Health Organ, 2007. 85(10): p. 783-90.
[19] Baqui, A.H., et al., *Rates, timing and causes of neonatal deaths in rural India: implications for neonatal health programmes.* Bull World Health Organ, 2006. 84(9): p. 706-13.
[20] Graneheim, U.H. and B. Lundman, *Qualitative content analysis in nursing research: concepts, procedures and measures to achieve trustworthiness.* Nurse Educ Today, 2004. 24(2): p. 105-12.
[21] Thaddeus, S. and D. Maine, *Too far to walk: maternal mortality in context.* Newsl Womens Glob Netw Reprod Rights, 1991(36): p. 22-4.
[22] Thaddeus, S. and D. Maine, *Too far to walk: maternal mortality in context.* Soc Sci Med, 1994. 38(8): p. 1091-110.
[23] Baqui, A.H., et al., *Newborn care in rural Uttar Pradesh.* Indian J Pediatr, 2007. 74(3): p. 241-7.
[24] World Health Organization. Maternal and Newborn Health / Safe Motherhood Unit., *Essential newborn care : report of a technical working group (Trieste, 25-29 April 1994)*1996, Geneva: World Health Organization. 19 p.
[25] Edmond, K.M., et al., *Delayed breastfeeding initiation increases risk of neonatal mortality.* Pediatrics, 2006. 117(3): p. e380-6.
[26] Engebretsen, I.M., et al., *Low adherence to exclusive breastfeeding in Eastern Uganda: a community-based cross-sectional study comparing dietary recall since birth with 24-hour recall.* BMC Pediatr, 2007. 7: p. 10.
[27] Hosseinpoor, A.R., et al., *Socioeconomic inequality in infant mortality in Iran and across its provinces.* Bull World Health Organ, 2005. 83(11): p. 837-44.
[28] Bryce, J., et al., *Reducing child mortality: can public health deliver?* Lancet, 2003. 362(9378): p. 159-64.
[29]Bhutta, Z.A., et al., *Delivering interventions to reduce the global burden of stillbirths: improving service supply and community demand.* BMC Pregnancy Childbirth, 2009. 9 Suppl 1: p. S7.
[30] Gabrysch, S. and O.M. Campbell, *Still too far to walk: literature review of the determinants of delivery service use.* BMC Pregnancy Childbirth, 2009. 9: p. 34.
[31] World Health Organization. Maternal and Newborn Health/Safe Motherhood., *Care of the umbilical cord : a review of the evidence*1998, Geneva: World Health Organization. 35 p.
[32] Mrisho, M., et al., *Understanding home-based neonatal care practice in rural southern Tanzania.* Trans R Soc Trop Med Hyg, 2008. 102(7): p. 669-78.
[33] Kesterton, A.J. and J. Cleland, *Neonatal care in rural Karnataka: healthy and harmful practices, the potential for change.* BMC Pregnancy Childbirth, 2009. 9: p. 20.
[34] Moran, A.C., et al., *Newborn care practices among slum dwellers in Dhaka, Bangladesh: a quantitative and qualitative exploratory study.* BMC Pregnancy Childbirth, 2009. 9: p. 54.

[35] Fikree, F.F., et al., *Newborn care practices in low socioeconomic settlements of Karachi, Pakistan.* Soc Sci Med, 2005. 60(5): p. 911-21.

[36] Sreeramareddy, C.T., et al., *Home delivery and newborn care practices among urban women in western Nepal: a questionnaire survey.* BMC Pregnancy Childbirth, 2006. 6: p. 27.

[37] Bhutta, Z.A., et al., *Interventions to address maternal, newborn, and child survival: what difference can integrated primary health care strategies make?* The Lancet, 2008. 372(9642): p. 972-989.

[38] Haines, A., S. Kuruvilla, and M. Borchert, *Bridging the implementation gap between knowledge and action for health.* Bull World Health Organ, 2004. 82(10): p. 724-31; discussion 732.

[39]Peterson, S., *Assessing the scale-up of child survival interventions.* Lancet, 2010. 375: p. 530-531.

[40] Victora, C.G., et al., *Context matters: interpreting impact findings in child survival evaluations.* Health Policy Plan, 2005. 20 Suppl 1: p. i18-i31.

[41] Mullany, L.C., G.L. Darmstadt, and J.M. Tielsch, *Safety and impact of chlorhexidine antisepsis interventions for improving neonatal health in developing countries.* Pediatr Infect Dis J, 2006. 25(8): p. 665-75.

[42] Mullany, L.C., et al., *A randomized controlled trial of the impact of chlorhexidine skin cleansing on bacterial colonization of hospital-born infants in Nepal.* Pediatr Infect Dis J, 2008. 27(6): p. 505-11.

[43] Lawn, J.E., K. Wilczynska-Ketende, and S.N. Cousens, *Estimating the causes of 4 million neonatal deaths in the year 2000.* Int J Epidemiol, 2006. 35(3): p. 706-18.

[44] Mbaruku, G., et al., *Perinatal audit using the 3-delays model in western Tanzania.* Int J Gynaecol Obstet, 2009. 106(1): p. 85-8.

[45] Bazzano, A.N., et al., *Beyond symptom recognition: care-seeking for ill newborns in rural Ghana.* Trop Med Int Health, 2008. 13(1): p. 123-8.

[46] Darmstadt, G.L., et al., *Household surveillance of severe neonatal illness by community health workers in Mirzapur, Bangladesh: coverage and compliance with referral.* Health Policy Plan, 2009.

[47] Rutebemberwa, E., et al., *Utilization of public or private health care providers by febrile children after user fee removal in Uganda.* Malar J, 2009. 8: p. 45.

[48] Rutebemberwa, E., et al., *Determinants of delay in care-seeking for febrile children in eastern Uganda.* Trop Med Int Health, 2009. 14(4): p. 472-9.

[49] Peterson, S., et al., *Coping with paediatric referral--Ugandan parents' experience.* Lancet, 2004. 363(9425): p. 1955-6.

[50] Duke, T., *Transport of seriously ill children: a neglected global issue.* Intensive Care Med, 2003. 29(9): p. 1414-6.

[51] Britto, J., et al., *Morbidity and severity of illness during interhospital transfer: impact of a specialised paediatric retrieval team.* BMJ, 1995. 311(7009): p. 836-9.

[52] Vos, G.D., et al., *Comparison of interhospital pediatric intensive care transport accompanied by a referring specialist or a specialist retrieval team.* Intensive Care Med, 2004. 30(2): p. 302-8.

[53] Eriksson, L., et al., *Evidence-based practice in neonatal health: knowledge among primary health care staff in northern Viet Nam.* Hum Resour Health, 2009. 7: p. 36.

[54] Opondo, C., et al., *Are hospitals prepared to support newborn survival? - an evaluation of eight first-referral level hospitals in Kenya*.* Trop Med Int Health, 2009.

[55] Hildenwall, H., et al., *Care-seeking in the development of severe community acquired pneumonia in Ugandan children.* Ann Trop Paediatr, 2009. 29(4): p. 281-9.

[56] Kiguli, J., et al., *Increasing access to quality health care for the poor: Community perceptions on quality care in Uganda.* Patient Prefer Adherence, 2009. 3: p. 77-85.

[57] Pariyo, G.W., et al., *Changes in utilization of health services among poor and rural residents in Uganda: are reforms benefitting the poor?* Int J Equity Health, 2009. 8: p. 39.
[58] Rutebemberwa, E., et al., *Use of drugs, perceived drug efficacy and preferred providers for febrile children: implications for home management of fever.* Malar J, 2009. 8: p. 131.
[59] Hildenwall, H., et al., *"I never had the money for blood testing" - caretakers' experiences of care-seeking for fatal childhood fevers in rural Uganda - a mixed methods study.* BMC Int Health Hum Rights, 2008. 8: p. 12.
[60] Kiwanuka, S.N., et al., *Access to and utilisation of health services for the poor in Uganda: a systematic review of available evidence.* Trans R Soc Trop Med Hyg, 2008. 102(11): p. 1067-74.
[61] Kallander, K., et al., *Delayed care seeking for fatal pneumonia in children aged under five years in Uganda: a case-series study.* Bull World Health Organ, 2008. 86(5): p. 332-8.
[62] Baqui, A.H., et al., *Effect of community-based newborn-care intervention package implemented through two service-delivery strategies in Sylhet district, Bangladesh: a cluster-randomised controlled trial.* Lancet, 2008. 371(9628): p. 1936-44.
[63] Haines, A., et al., *Achieving child survival goals: potential contribution of community health workers.* Lancet, 2007. 369(9579): p. 2121-31.
[64] Baqui, A.H., et al., *Effectiveness of home-based management of newborn infections by community health workers in rural Bangladesh.* Pediatr Infect Dis J, 2009. 28(4): p. 304-10.
[65] Kumar, V., et al., *Effect of community-based behaviour change management on neonatal mortality in Shivgarh, Uttar Pradesh, India: a cluster-randomised controlled trial.* Lancet, 2008. 372(9644): p. 1151-62.
[66] Darmstadt, G.L., et al., *Introduction of community-based skin-to-skin care in rural Uttar Pradesh, India.* J Perinatol, 2006. 26(10): p. 597-604.
[67] Waiswa, P., et al., *Acceptability of evidence-based neonatal care practices in rural Uganda - implications for programming.* BMC Pregnancy Childbirth, 2008. 8: p. 21.
[68] Pattinson, R., et al., *Perinatal mortality audit: Counting, accountability, and overcoming challenges in scaling up in low- and middle-income countries.* Int J Gynaecol Obstet, 2009.
[69] Wall, S.N., et al., *Neonatal resuscitation in low-resource settings: What, who, and how to overcome challenges to scale up?* Int J Gynaecol Obstet, 2009.
[70] Bhutta, Z.A., et al., *Management of newborn infections in primary care settings: a review of the evidence and implications for policy?* Pediatr Infect Dis J, 2009. 28(1 Suppl): p. S22-30.
[71] Reyes H, P.-C.R., Salmeron J, Tome P, Guiscafre´ H, Gutierrez G *Infant mortality due to acute respiratory infections: the influence of primary care processes.* Health Policy Planning 1997. 12: p. 214-223.
[72] Tolhurst, R., et al., *'I don't want all my babies to go to the grave': perceptions of preterm birth in Southern Malawi.* Midwifery, 2008. 24(1): p. 83-98.
[73] UBOS, *Demographic and Health Survey 2006.*, U.B.o.S.a. MACRO/USAID, Editor 2006: Kampala.
[74] Wamani, H., et al., *Infant and young child feeding in western Uganda: knowledge, practices and socio-economic correlates.* J Trop Pediatr, 2005. 51(6): p. 356-61.
[75] Winikoff, B. and V.H. Laukaran, *Breast feeding and bottle feeding controversies in the developing world: evidence from a study in four countries.* Soc Sci Med, 1989. 29(7): p. 859-68.
[76] Howard, C., et al., *Office prenatal formula advertising and its effect on breast-feeding patterns.* Obstet Gynecol, 2000. 95(2): p. 296-303.
[77] Dennis, C.L., *Breastfeeding initiation and duration: a 1990-2000 literature review.* J Obstet Gynecol Neonatal Nurs, 2002. 31(1): p. 12-32.

3

Recent Advances in Neonatal Gastroenterology and Neonatal Nutrition

Shripad Rao, Madhur Ravikumara, Gemma McLeod and Karen Simmer
Centre for Neonatal Research and Education, The University of Western Australia, Neonatology Clinical Care Unit and the Department of Gastroenterology, King Edward Memorial Hospital and Princess Margaret Hospital, Perth, Australia

1. Introduction

Nutrition plays an important role in achieving optimal growth and development of the high risk neonate. Recent developments have shown that aggressive parenteral nutrition defined as relatively high amounts of parenteral protein and lipid commencing on the first day of life reduces the incidence of ex-utero growth retardation (EUGR) and associated morbidities.

For preterm infants, early minimal enteral feed and a standardised feeding regime have improved clinical outcomes. Probiotics appear useful in further reducing the incidence of necrotizing enterocolitis (NEC).

Short-gut syndrome is not infrequent after NEC and fish oil lipid emulsions are useful in the prevention and treatment of intestinal failure-associated liver disease (IFALD).

Use of preformed silos has been shown to improve the outcomes of gastroschisis by decreasing the risk of abdominal compartment syndrome and iatrogenic gut ischemia.

Until recently, neonatal haemochromatosis was considered uniformly fatal disease and only curative treatment was liver transplantation. Exchange transfusion and intravenous immunoglobulin therapy are emerging as potentially curative strategies for this condition.

High index of suspicion and early diagnosis and management of malrotation is highly essential to prevent the dreaded complication of volvulus with intestinal gangrene.

The WHO 2006 growth charts are useful in monitoring the subsequent growth term infants and avoid over-diagnosis of growth failure and under-diagnosis of obesity. These growth charts also have the potential of being useful in monitoring the growth of preterm infants after post-conceptional age of 40 weeks.

In this chapter, we have reviewed all these recent advances and potentially better practices which most likely will help improve the outcomes of high risk neonates.

2. Recent developments in nutrition for preterm infants

Growth retardation after preterm birth or EUGR is defined as discharge weight less than the 10th percentile of intra-uterine growth expectation. The risk of EUGR increases with decreasing gestational age and birth weight. Dusick et al (Dusick et al. 2003) using NICHD network (National Institute of Child and Human Development) reported that nearly 100% of very low birth weight (501 - 1500g) infants have growth failure at 36 weeks post-conceptional age (PCA). They also reported that 40% were still less than the 10th percentile for weight at 18 months of age.

Impaired growth during and after discharge from hospital is associated with increased neurodevelopmental problem in infancy and early childhood(Latal-Hajnal et al. 2003, Ehrenkranz et al. 2006). Current consensus is that the neonatologists should be focused on improving the early nutrient management of these infants, allowing them to reach an adequate growth rate (at least 18-20 g/kg/d), thereby avoiding the need of a late un-physiological catch-up growth(Fanaro 2010). Hence, nutritional guidelines have been revised with the aim of reducing EUGR and sequalae (Tsang R et al. 2005). The revised nutritional recommendations theoretically should result in body composition similar to a healthy fetus that has less body fat than most preterm infants currently have at term. The new guidelines recommend protein intakes of 3.5 to 4.5g/kg/day and up to 130 – 150 kcal/kg/day.

Once EUGR occurs, excessive catch up growth may lead to increased adiposity and insulin resistance and metabolic syndrome later in life (Yeung 2006, Morrison et al. 2010). This has led to a dilemma after discharge: whether to aim for better nutrition to achieve improved neurodevelopmental outcomes, which may come at a cost of early-onset obesity and diabetes (Ong 2007).

A recent randomised trial has shown that catch-up growth if achieved with optimal nutrition may not lead to excessive central adiposity(Cooke et al. 2010). Preterm infants with a GA <34 wk and a birth weight of <1750 g were randomized immediately before hospital discharge to be fed with a nutrient-enriched formula or a standard formula for 6 months. They found that more rapid and more complete "catch-up," was noted in infants fed with the nutrient-enriched formula. This "catch-up" was due to increased fat free mass and fat accretion on the legs rather than central adiposity measured by DEXA.

The results of this RCT provide some reassurance that catch up growth and hence improved neurodevelopmental outcomes may be achievable without paying the price of increased risk of obesity, diabetes and hypertension. Similar studies and long term follow up are desirable to gain further knowledge in this area.

2.1 Parenteral nutrition

In extremely preterm infants, at least 1.5g/kg/day of protein is required to prevent negative nitrogen balance and 3.5g/kg/day to achieve positive balance (fetal equivalent) . It has been calculated that if a 26 week gestation infant receives only glucose, he will have a 25% deficit of body protein by 1 week of age (Dusick et al. 2003). There is evidence from randomised controlled trials that an aggressive nutritional regime in the early weeks can minimise the large protein deficit most ELBW babies incur, and reduce the rate of extra-uterine growth retardation (Wilson et al. 1997, Dinerstein et al. 2006). Starting parenteral nutrition on day 1 and providing at least 3g/kg/day amino acids by day 5 will reduce the incidence of EUGR, improve nitrogen retention and maintain amino acids within the fetal reference range(Poindexter et al. 2006, te Braake et al. 2007). Extremely low birth weight (ELBW) infants require 70 kcal/kg/d for basal metabolic rate. Their glucose requirement is 8-12 mg/kg/min (45-56 cal) with the balance of non-protein cal given as intravenous lipid. Early lipid (day 2-4), up to 3g/kg/d (27cal/kg/d) is well tolerated with no documented adverse effects(Simmer and Rao 2005). The lipid emulsion currently used in Australia is based on soybean oil and is rich in essential fatty acids (EFA, 60%). Alternative lipid emulsions with a mixture of olive, and soybean oil are available commercially in some countries. Advantages of the new blends include lower EFA content and more alpha tocopherol which may result in improved ability to synthesise longer chain metabolites which are the precursors of eicosanoids, reduced lipid peroxidation and oxidative stress, and attenuation of immunosuppressive effects linked to LA. More recently, fish-oil based emulsions have been introduced to prevent and treat parenteral-nutrition induced cholestasis, and to provide preformed DHA. Lipid emulsions available for neonatal parenteral nutrition are reviewed by Deshpande & Simmer (2011) (Deshpande and Simmer 2011).

2.2 Enteral nutrition

Minimal enteral feeds, even for very immature infants, should be started in the first few days at 5 - 10mls/kg/day of human milk. The earlier that enteral feeds are commenced, the earlier full enteral feeds are achieved. Early full enteral feeds is associated with reduced late onset sepsis with no increase in NEC (Ronnestad et al. 2005, Kennedy et al. 2000). Mother's own milk (MOM) is the feed of choice as benefits include improved intelligence, lower infection rates and less NEC (Vohr et al. 2006, Schanler 2001).

Early milk has higher content of nutritional and immunological factors and should be used first. Freezing the milk will greatly reduce the viral CMV load and therefore risk of CMV transmission from unpasteurised milk. If inadequate MOM available, pasteurised donor human milk (PDHM) is preferred to artificial formula. All human milk will require fortification for preterm infants to meet recommended nutritional intakes for optimal growth. Feeds are usually fortified after full enteral feeds are tolerated because of possibility that the higher osmolality of fortified milk may contribute to NEC. Commercial fortifiers contain protein, energy, calcium, phosphate, sodium, minerals and vitamins and are well tolerated by most preterm infants. If MOM and PDHM are unavailable, preterm infants should be fed preterm formula rather than term formula until discharge, as it is tailored to meet the nutritional needs of preterm infants. There is concern that cows' milk protein is a risk factor for NEC and for allergic disease in childhood (Berg et al. 2010, von Berg et al. 2008) and there are commercial fortifiers and preterm formula available that do not contain intact cows' milk protein.

2.3 Human Milk Banks (HMBs)

For preterm infants PDHM reduces the incidence of NEC four fold and improves feed tolerance(Quigley et al. 2007). This may be associated with reduced days of parental nutrition and earlier discharge from hospital. Pasteurisation reduces the protective effects of human milk but feeding PDHM is still associated with a lower incidence of infections than feeding formula.

Most informal HMBs closed in the 1980's due to the discovery that the HIV virus could be transmitted through breastfeeding. Many countries have now re-established human milk banking with comprehensive risk management processes, most HMBs provide PDHM for preterm infants while in hospital. In Australia, the HMB runs by the code of good manufacturing practices (blood and tissues) and models risk management on codex HACCP (Hazard Analysis Critical Control Point) requirements(Hartmann et al. 2007). Parental consent for PDHM is obtained by lactation consultants to ensure full support of breastfeeding.

2.4 High dose supplements

Long chain polyunsaturated fatty acids (LCPUFA) especially docosahexaenoic acid (DHA) may be important for optimal neurological development of preterm infants. The Cochrane Review of LCPUFA supplementation of formula for preterm infants found that there was little evidence to support a benefit but a suggestion but supplementation was usually low dose as it was aimed at breast milk equivalence (0.2-0.5% DHA) (Schulzke et al. 2011). Makrides et al (2009) randomised 657 infants < 33 weeks gestation to high dose DHA, (approximately 1% DHA aimed at *in utero* supply) by supplementing lactating mothers to increase breast milk DHA (average breast milk levels). Bayley mental developmental index was higher at 18 months (girls only) and there was less developmental delay (all infants) especially in the < 1250 g subgroup, with high dose DHA supplementation compared with low-moderate dose (0.3% DHA). (Makrides et al. 2009).

Vitamin A is required for normal lung growth and meta-analysis of clinical trials suggests that Vitamin A supplementation is associated with reduction in death and chronic lung disease in preterm infants. The optimal dose for extremely low birth weight infants (<1kg) appears to be 5000 IU IM three times weekly for four weeks (Darlow and Graham 2007). Vitamin A delivery from parenteral nutrition is better if added to lipid emulsion.

Probiotic supplementation of VLBW infants reduces death and NEC (Deshpande et al. 2010). Sourcing a preparation is challenging in most countries. On-line evidence-based guidelines for the use of probiotics in preterm infants are available(Deshpande et al. 2011).

In summary, avoidance of postnatal growth retardation, early parenteral nutrition with fish/olive oil based lipid emulsions, early enteral feeding with human milk, supplementation with DHA, vitamin A and probiotics are potentially best practices to achieve optimal clinical outcomes after preterm birth.

3. Intrauterine growth restriction

3.1 Definition and diagnosis

Birth weight is determined by gestational age at time of delivery and by fetal growth rate (5 g/d at 14-15 wk gestation; 10 g/d at 20 w gestation; 30-35 g/d at 32-34 w gestation) (Williams et al. 1982)) and its classification describes an infant's birth weight relative to a population reference. In statistical terms, small for gestational age (SGA) denotes a birth weight two standard deviations (SD) below the median birth weight for gestational age (GA). Although <2 SD below the median approximates the 2.3rd percentile(De Curtis and Rigo 2004), and may be a more relevant cutoff for indicating perinatal risk, neonates with a birth weight below the 10th percentile for GA are commonly classified as SGA. The term SGA is often used synonymously with intrauterine growth restriction (IUGR), largely because of the difficulties associated with diagnosing IUGR. However, the SGA infant population is a heterogeneous group, with some being constitutionally small, without any underlying pathology (80-85%) whilst others have demonstrated IUGR, implying conceptually, that genetically determined growth potential has not been achieved *in utero*(Breeze and Lees 2007, Levene et al. 2000). Distinction between a healthy small fetus and one with IUGR can be facilitated by ultrasound examination to detect chromosomal abnormality, amniotic fluid volume changes, serial fetal growth symmetry monitoring and Doppler studies. Utilising customised standards for fetal growth and birth weight that adjust for maternal variables of height, weight, parity and ethnic group, may further improve the accurate detection of IUGR(Figueras and Gardosi 2011). The aim of identifying IUGR is to reduce associated perinatal morbidity and mortality, primarily by optimising the timing and mode of delivery of the growth restricted fetus.

3.2 Incidence and aetiology

The study of IUGR has been thwarted by ambiguous terminology and a lack of uniform standards and diagnostic criteria. Most recently this ambiguity has been demonstrated by Olsen et al.(2010). These investigators compared new intrauterine growth curves based on US data collected from 391 681 racially diverse infants to the commonly used Lubchenco curves(Lubchenco et al. 1963) and found that the SGA classifications differed significantly for each gestational age ($p<0.0001$), with the Lubchenco curves underestimating the percentage of infants who were SGA. Similarly, Goldenberg et al(1989) compared 13 different standards from different populations and geographic areas and found a discrepancy of more than 500 g between GA-specific cut-off values used by different investigators to define IUGR. These anomalies affect the accuracy of incidence data. Nevertheless, IUGR is thought to affect 7-15% of all pregnancies worldwide(Alisi et al. 2011), and a substantial proportion of IUGR fetuses are delivered preterm. IUGR is not a specific disease entity, but rather, is related to medical conditions compromising (i) placental circulation and efficiency (e.g. placental praevia, placental insufficiency and toxaemia of pregnanacy), (ii) fetal growth and development (e.g. chromosomal disorders, congenital malformations, multiple gestations and infection) and/or (iii) maternal health and nutrition (e.g. pregnancy induced hypertension, maternal hypoxia, vascular and renal disease, substance abuse and malnutrition)(Resnik 2002). The timing of the insult determines whether IUGR is symmetrical or asymmetrical, an outcome linked predominantly to the three phases of fetal growth (cellular hyperplasia: first 16 weeks of gestation; concomitant hyperplasia and hypertrophy: 16-32 weeks gestation; and cellular hypertrophy: 32 weeks to term). Early onset IUGR, arising from severe maternal vascular disease, infection (notably TORCH infections: toxoplasmosis, rubella, cytomegalovirus, varicella, HIV) and chromosomal or structural abnormalities such as cardiac and renal conditions, give rise to small infants with hypoplasia, who display symmetrical growth reductions in weight, length and head circumference (no head-sparing effect) and have a normal ponderal index (PI) [$PI = (\text{birth weight (g)}/\text{Length (cm)}^3)*100$; normal PI is ≥ 2.41; low PI is <2.41]. These infants are unable to achieve their genetically determined growth potential. Later onset of IUGR results from utero-placental disorders and maternal factors leading to impaired delivery of oxygen and nutrients from the placenta. These factors come into play at different times and to varying degrees of severity during pregnancy, but generally, later onset IUGR results in asymmetric growth characterized by a relatively greater decrease in abdominal size (subcutaneous fat and liver volume), low PI, and sparing of head and length(Levene et al. 2000) with potential for some catch up growth.

3.3 Pathophysiology

Compared to gestational-age matched peers, those with IUGR are at higher risk of morbidity and mortality(Damodaram et al. 2011), particularly if growth restriction is severe(Vossbeck et al. 2001, Wienerroither et al. 2001) and delivery is very preterm(Bernstein et al. 2000). The fetus chronically deprived of oxygen and substrates is at increased risk of stillbirth, fetal distress, congenital malformation, meconium aspiration, cord compression, premature rupture of membranes and preterm birth. Neonatal death, asphyxia, hypoglycaemia, meconium aspiration syndrome, polycythaemia, hyperviscosity, hypothermia, infection, pulmonary haemorrhage and transient neonatal hpyperglycaemia are anticipated features of the growth-restricted neonate(Damodaram et al. 2011, Levene et al. 2000). The IUGR preterm infant is also at increased risk of developing necrotizing enterocolitis and respiratory distress syndrome(Bernstein et al. 2000), and may demonstrate continued impaired growth and developmental delay(Bhide 2011, Levene et al.. 2000). IUGR is also associated in later life with features of the metabolic syndrome, including insulin resistance, hypertension, impaired glucose tolerance(Barker 2004) and very recently, nonalcoholic fatty liver disease(Alisi et al. 2011). The fetal adaptations to inadequate nutrition and subsequent IUGR that produce these long-term outcomes are incompletely understood but relate to fetal glucose and fuel metabolism. The adaptations have apparent survival value for the fetus by encouraging efficient glucose and energy utilization, by reducing uptake of amino acids for growth, by reducing production of anabolic hormone, and by increasing glucose supply to vital organs. In the short-term, these survival-motivated adaptations result in asymmetrical growth with some head and length sparing but if these adaptive mechanisms are prolonged or if their onset is more easily inducible in later life, the potential may exist for energy uptake beyond metabolic capacity(Thorn et al. 2011). The adverse outcomes of mismatched pre- and postnatal nutrition and catch up growth have been well demonstrated in animal models (Cleal et al. 2007, Ozanne and Hales 2004).

3.4 Management

The current treatment for IUGR is delivery and the main considerations need to be timing and mode of delivery, balancing the risk of neonatal morbidity with continued exposure to a stressful intrauterine environment. Careful monitoring of fetal and uteroplacental function with tests such as serial ultrasound scans, Doppler assessment of umbilical flow and cardiac monitoring will assist in determining optimal delivery time. Admission to a special care nursery (SCN) for observation is necessary for the severely growth restricted infant. It is worth noting that the IUGR phenotype includes decreased pancreatic development and insulin secretion capacity, as well as an up-regulated capacity for glucose uptake and a decreased capacity for synthesising protein for growth(Hay 2008). As Hay(2008) suggests, this could mean that equal rates of amino acids infused into a chronically IUGR infant may not translate to the same increase in growth as that observed in the healthy fetus born preterm and further, that attempts to infuse higher rates of intravenous glucose may produce both lactic acidosis and lipogenesis more readily in the IUGR infant than in the healthy preterm infant. Nutrition recommendations that specifically target IUGR preterm infants are lacking. Feeding regimes for IUGR preterm infants are usually similar to those who are appropriately grown, with some caution as feeds are progressed because of increased risk of NEC. Attention should be given to providing adequate nourishment for the

IUGR preterm infant from birth so that percentiles are at least maintained and so that extrauterine growth is of proportionate composition to that of the age-matched fetus.

3.5 Future research directions

Future research should focus on developing nutrition recommendations and feeding strategies specific for IUGR preterm infants.

Further investigation of the quality of catch up growth achieved by asymmetrically grown IUGR preterm infants in response to macronutrient and energy intakes and implications of catch up growth.

Further elucidation of the mechanisms underlying fetal and postnatal adaptation to IUGR and the impact of these adaptations on long-term health.

Standardisation of IUGR definition, diagnostic tools and method of diagnosis.

4. Growth monitoring of preterm infants during NICU stay and post discharge

Growth monitoring of preterm neonates is particularly important in the context of evidence that postnatal growth restriction is associated with long term adverse neuro-developmental outcomes (Ehrenkranz et al. 2006, Shah et al. 2006, Casey et al. 2006, Latal-Hajnal et al. 2003). Careful growth monitoring while in, and after discharge from, NICU has the potential to improve long term outcomes.

4.1 Types of growth curves currently available for use in preterm infants

A 'standard' chart represents the ideal healthy growth of a population and hence is of prescriptive nature. A 'reference' chart describes the population without making claims about the health of its sample and hence is descriptive in nature. At present, there are no standard growth charts for preterm infants.

4.2 Intra uterine growth curves

The American Academy of Pediatrics('American Academy of Pediatrics Committee on Nutrition: Nutritional needs of low-birth-weight infants' 1985) and Canadian Pediatric society('Nutrient needs and feeding of premature infants. Nutrition Committee, Canadian Paediatric Society' 1995) recommend intra uterine growth rates as the ideal growth of preterm infants. There are more than 25 studies reporting on such 'intrauterine growth charts'. These have been best summarized by Karna et al (Karna et al. 2005). Lubchenko 1963(Lubchenco et al. 1963) and Babson/Benda1976 (Babson and Benda 1976) charts are commonly used in many neonatal units around the world. Fenton et al(Fenton 2003) updated the Babson and Benda growth curves to develop contemporary 'intrauterine growth curves'. Using preset criteria, three recent large population based surveys of birth weight for gestational age were identified. The Canadian study by Kramer(Kramer et al. 2001) which had a sample size of 676,605 infants delivered between 22 to 43 weeks was used for updating the intrauterine weight section. Two large studies, one from Sweden(Niklasson et al. 1991) and one from Australia(Beeby et al. 1996) were used to update the intrauterine head circumference and length section. The data were averaged together using a weighted average based on total sample size to derive the 3rd, 10th, 50th, 95th and 97th percentiles and create one growth chart. CDC 2000 growth charts were used to generate the growth curves from corrected gestation of 40 weeks onwards.

The Fenton chart appears to be useful in monitoring the growth of preterm infants during their NICU stay till they reach corrected gestation of 40 weeks. It is used by many North American, European and Australian centres. Recently Olsen et al have published new intrauterine growth curves based on United States data(Olsen et al. 2010).

The inherent problem with intrauterine growth charts is that, even though they are called "intrauterine" charts, they are in fact cross sectional data derived from anthropometry measured at birth on preterm infants delivered at various gestations. It is well known that fetuses delivered prematurely may not have reached full growth potential due various maternal/fetal morbidities and hence do not reflect the "ideal" growth. Also, these charts do not take into consideration, the normal 5-8% weight loss that occurs in healthy preterm infants in the first week of life.

4.3 'Fetal growth curves'

Strictly speaking, only charts derived from longitudinal studies should be called growth charts, growth being a process extended over time(Bertino et al. 2007). Hence it may appear logical that ideal 'intrauterine growth charts' should be derived from serial and longitudinal assessment of physical parameters of weight, length and head circumference using fetal ultrasound technique(Johnsen et al. 2006). However, the drawback of this method is that fetal ultrasound is not very accurate in predicting the fetal weight. A systematic review(Chauhan et al. 2005) which analysed data from 58 articles over 28 years found wide variability in diagnostic accuracy of ultrasound examination in predicting the fetal weight. Another systematic review(Dudley 2005) concluded that the accuracy of estimated fetal weight using fetal ultrasound is compromised by large intra- and inter-observer variability. Also, maternal morbidities can result in fetal growth restriction, which in turn can result in non- ideal growth charts. In view of such limitations, fetal weight curves derived from the currently available ultrasound technology may not be appropriate for use as ideal postnatal growth of preterm infants.

4.4 Reference' Growth charts

Many reference charts that describe the actual longitudinal growth of preterm infants during the course of their stay in the NICU have been published (Diekmann et al. 2005, Bertino et al. 2006). If these reference charts are used to monitor the ongoing growth of preterm infants, extra-uterine growth retardation would be considered as normal. Hence they may not be ideal for monitoring the growth of preterm infants. However, these charts give an idea of what can be achieved with the available resources and limits set by the morbidities of prematurity and can be used compare the growth of preterm infants between different units.

4.5 A note of caution regarding the use of intra uterine growth charts

Intra uterine growth charts may appear idealistic goals, but one needs to decide if it is really feasible and safe to attain those parameters. Attempts to promote physical growth by aggressive enteral and parenteral nutrition have the potential to harm the sick preterm infant. Rapid increase in enteral feeding is a known risk factor for NEC (Berseth et al. 2003). In ELBW infants, high fluid intake associated with less weight loss during the first 10 days of life is associated with an increased risk of death and BPD (Oh et al. 2005, Wadhawan et al. 2007). In addition excessive catch up growth may result in adverse cardiovascular outcomes later in life. Finken et al(Finken et al. 2006) and Euser etal(Euser et al. 2005) found that in subjects born very preterm, rapid weight gain in infancy was associated with a trend towards higher insulin levels at 19 years. They also concluded that rapid weight gain in both infancy and early childhood is a risk factor for adult adiposity and obesity. Similar concerns have been raised by other investigators (Ekelund et al. 2006, Singhal et al. 2007).

4.6 Growth charts to monitor preterm infants from post-conceptional age of 40 weeks into early childhood

Until recently, many countries used the growth charts released by Centers for Disease Control and Prevention (CDC 2000) for monitoring the growth of term infants and children. The same charts are usually used for ongoing growth monitoring of preterm infants after reaching a corrected gestational age of 40 weeks. The inherent problem with such charts is that they represent the actual existing growth patterns instead of recommended standards.

To resolve this problem inherent with 'reference' charts, WHO has recently released new 'Standard' growth charts for term infants and children(WHO 2006). The WHO multicentre growth reference study (MGRS), was conducted between 1997 and 2003 in 6 countries from diverse geographical regions: Brazil, Ghana, India, Norway, Oman and the United States. The study combined a longitudinal follow-up of 882 infants from birth to 24 months with a cross-sectional component of 6669 children aged 18-71 months. The study populations lived in socioeconomic conditions favourable to growth. The individual inclusion criteria for the longitudinal component were: no known health or environmental constraints to growth, mothers willing to follow MGRS feeding recommendations (i.e. exclusive or predominant breastfeeding for at least 4 months, introduction of complementary foods by 6 months of age and continued breastfeeding to at least 12 months of age), no maternal smoking before and after delivery, single-term birth and absence of significant morbidity. The eligibility criteria for the cross-sectional component were the same as those for the longitudinal component with the exception of infant feeding practices. A minimum of 3 months of any breastfeeding was required for participants in the study's cross-sectional component. Weight-for-age, length/height-for-age, weight-for-length/height and body mass index-for-age percentile and Z-score values were generated for boys and girls aged 0-60 months. The pooled sample from the 6 participating countries allowed the development of a truly international reference. The standards explicitly identify breastfeeding as the biological norm and establish the breastfed child as the normative model for growth and development. They also demonstrate that healthy children from around the world who are raised in healthy environments and follow recommended feeding practices have strikingly similar patterns of growth. These charts are recommendations for how children should grow. More than 100 countries including UK, USA, Canada and New Zealand have started using the WHO growth charts for full term infants. The full set of tables and charts are available on the WHO website (*www.who.int/childgrowth/en*) together with tools such as software and training materials.

In the absence of other ideal growth charts, it may be reasonable to use these WHO growth charts to monitor the ongoing growth of preterm infants after reaching post-conceptional age of 40 weeks.

4.7 Future research

As discussed above, neither "intrauterine growth charts", "fetal growth charts" nor "postnatal growth charts" are suitable for monitoring the growth of preterm infants till they become term. Similarly, CDC 2000 and WHO 2006 growth charts are also not ideal for monitoring the growth of ex-preterm infants.

In order to establish normative growth charts, the Inter Growth 21st study by the International Fetal and Newborn Growth Consortium has commenced ('http://www.intergrowth21.org.uk/' Accessed 18 September, 2011). The study aims to recruit 4500 healthy women aged 18-35, who had regular menstrual cycles and conceived spontaneously and do not have major health issues and practice healthy lifestyles. Study participant women are recruited from 9 countries across five continents. They undergo 6 scans in addition to the initial dating scans. They are scheduled at 5 weekly intervals: 14-18 weeks, 19-23 weeks, 24-28 weeks, 29-33weeks, 34-38 weeks and 39-42 weeks. Apart from the additional scans, they receive the standardized antenatal care. Based on expected 9% rate of prematurity, it is expected that around 360 infants would be born to these mothers (26-37 weeks gestation). Their longitudinal growth will be monitored for 8 months. This would include measuring weight, length and head circumference every 2 weeks for the first eight weeks and then monthly until eight months after birth. Those suffering from death or serious morbidities of prematurity such as NEC will be excluded. This will study will enable the derivation of prescriptive intrauterine growth curves as well as postnatal growth curves from a diverse population across five continents.

In summary:

1. Intra uterine growth curves, even though are not ideal, are recommended by leading professional paediatric organisations. In the absence of better charts, they are to be used for monitoring the growth of preterm infants.
2. Postnatal growth curves describe the actual growth and hence are descriptive rather than prescriptive. They are not suitable for monitoring the growth of preterm infants.
3. The aim when caring for preterm infants is to at least match the growth velocity of published best postnatal growth curves and strive towards reaching ideal growth velocities of intrauterine growth curves.
4. Due to improvements in management of sick preterm infants, the growth of these infants in 1990 and 2000s is different from those of previous years. Hence it is preferable to use the growth curves developed based on preterm infants born after 1990.
5. The Fenton chart which has updated the Babson and Benda's chart with data from very large sample size of preterm infants born in the last two decades appears to be suitable for monitoring growth of preterm infants during their stay in the neonatal units.
6. Once a post-conceptional age of 40 weeks is reached, the recently released WHO growth curves can be used to monitor their ongoing growth.
7. While aiming for achieving intrauterine growth velocities in postnatal life, one should not lose sight of the potential short term adverse effects of aggressive nutrition and long term adverse effects of excessive catch up growth.

The currently ongoing "Intergrowth-21st study" has the potential to overcome the deficiencies of all the existing growth curves and will enable the establishment of prescriptive growth curves for monitoring the growth of preterm infants during and beyond their NICU stay into early childhood.

5. Probiotics for the prevention of necrotizing enterocolitis

Necrotizing enterocolitis is a devastating condition in preterm and very low birth weight neonates and carries significant mortality and morbidity (Berrington et al. 2011). Survivors of NEC suffer from significant adverse neurodevelopmental outcomes(Schulzke et al. 2007).

The commonly employed strategies for its prevention are standardised feeding regimen, slow initiation and progression of enteral feeds and preferential use of breast milk (Morgan et al. 2011). In spite of these measures, NEC continues to occur and the latest figures suggest that the incidence in extremely low gestational age neonates is around 11%(Stoll et al. 2010).

Gastro-intestinal colonisation by pathogenic bacteria is one of the important factors in the pathogenesis of necrotising enterocolitis(Claud and Walker 2001).

Probiotics are defined as live microbial supplements that colonise the gut while providing benefits to the host(Millar et al. 2003). Supplementation with probiotic organisms have been shown to replace the pathogenic bacteria from the intestines by the normal healthy flora. This rationale lead to the conduct of randomised controlled trials, majority of which have consistently shown that probiotic supplementation reduces the incidence of severe necrotising enterocolitis (≥stage 2). Our meta analysis on this subject estimated a significantly lower risk of NEC in the probiotic group (relative risk [RR]: 0.35 [95% confidence interval (CI): 0.23–0.55]; $P < .00001$)(Deshpande et al. 2010). We concluded that further placebo controlled RCTs may not be necessary and probiotic supplementation should be offered routinely for all preterm infants. The updated Cochrane review also expressed similar sentiments (Alfaleh et al. 2011). However, others still are skeptical and advocate caution (Soll 2010, Neu and Shuster 2010) while others feel the evidence is enough to warrant routine use (Tarnow-Mordi et al. 2010, Barrington 2011)

Further to this, our group has published evidence based guidelines for the administration of probiotics in preterm infants for those who believe in probiotic supplementation (Deshpande et al. 2011). Our suggestions for the routine administration of probiotics for preterm infants (≤ 34 weeks) are as follows:

a. Selection of strains: Combination containing Lactobacillus and at least one Bifidobacterium species is preferable. Lactobacillus GG alone may not be effective. Dose: 3×10^9 organisms per day, preferably in a single dose
b. When to commence: When the neonate is ready for enteral feeds, preferably within first 7 days of life.
c. How long to continue: At least until 35 weeks corrected age, or discharge.
d. When to stop: Stopping the supplementation during an acute illness such as sepsis, NEC or perinatal asphyxia may be safe.

A very important step is to find a good quality product meeting the strict criteria of individual countries' drug administration bodies is essential.

6. Neonatal short bowel syndrome

Short-bowel syndrome (SBS), which results from surgical resection or congenital defect (Goulet and Ruemmele 2006, O'Keefe et al. 2006) is a sub category of intestinal failure. Intestinal failure is defined as intrinsic bowel disease resulting in an inability to sustain growth, hydration and electrolyte homeostasis unless parenteral nutrition is provided. Intestinal failure results from intestinal obstruction, dysmotility, surgical resection, congenital defects, or disease-associated loss of absorption and is characterized by the inability to maintain protein-energy, fluid, electrolyte, or micronutrient balance. The Canadian Association of Pediatric Surgeons defines SBS as the need for parenteral nutrition greater than 42 days after bowel resection or a residual small bowel length of less than 25% expected for gestational age (Wales et al. 2005). Normal small bowel length increases from 1145 cm between 19 and 27 weeks of gestation through to 172 cm between 27 and 35 weeks of gestation to a length of 248 cm in neonates greater than 35 weeks of gestation (Touloukian and Smith 1983). At 1 year of age, small bowel length is approximately 380 cm (Touloukian and Smith 1983).

The primary aetiologies of SBS in neonatal population are: Necrotizing enterocolitis, intestinal atresias, gastroschisis, malrotation with volvulus, and Hirschprung's disease that extends into the small bowel(Gutierrez et al. 2011).

The principles of management involve multidisciplinary approach focused on nutritional, pharmacologic, and surgical interventions that is directed to achieve maximal gut adaptation and full enteral nutrition while minimizing the complications of PN therapy.

Providing nutrition parenterally is the essential until the gut adaptation is complete and full enteral feeds are tolerated to maintain growth, hydration and electrolyte homeostasis Adequate Glucose, amino acids, lipids and micronutrients should be administered to optimize growth and development. Generally it is recommended that the amount of glucose not to exceed 18g/kg body weight/day(Koletzko et al. 2008), which is shown to be the maximum rate of glucose utilisation. Excessive glucose infusion is considered to be one of the contributing factor for the development of intestinal failure associated liver disease (IFALD).

Lipids are an important source of energy, essential fatty acids and fat soluble vitamins and an essential component of any parenteral nutrition (PN) regimen. Soya bean based lipid emulsions are the commonly used lipid source in most PN solutions. There is increasing evidence that soya bean based lipid emulsions can result in liver disease due to the pro-inflammatory nature of the w-6 fatty acids. Fish oil based lipid emulsions are rich in w-3 fatty acids which are anti inflammatory and have been shown to be protective against IFLAD and hence are preferred in patients with SBS, especially in those who are likely to need long term PN support(Fallon et al. 2010, Lilja et al. 2011).

Low serum bicarbonate and sodium levels are common in patients with SBS due to increased fecal or stoma loss. The former may be managed by increasing acetate in the PN or enteral supplementation of sodium bicarbonate as tolerated. An important but often neglected complication is chronic body sodium depletion in babies with short gut. Prolonged sodium losses and inadequate supplementation leads to growth failure in neonates. Serum sodium levels may be maintained in the normal range despite inadequate supplementation due to compensatory hyperaldosteronism. Adequate sodium should be administered in the PN or enterally to maintain urinary sodium of > 30meq/l and sodium/potassium ratio of atleast 1 (Kocoshis 2010).

It is important to commence enteral feeds as soon as feasible to prevent complications of TPN and to enable intestinal growth and adaptation. A recent systematic review found very limited number high quality studies addressing the issue of enteral nutrition in infants and children with SBS (Olieman et al. 2010). Hence most of the recommendations are expert opinions or consensus based:

a. Enteral nutrition should be initiated as soon as possible (ie, a few days after bowel resection). Volumes should be gradually increased by 1 mL/hr twice a week. Tolerance of new volumes can be assessed by (a) vomiting (more than three times per day/more than 20% of their daily enteral intake is extensive and indicates intolerance) and (b) quantity and consistency of stool, pH, and sugar reduction of stool. Enteral feeds could be advanced as long as stool or stomal output is <2 mL/kg/h. Because not all enterally administered calories will be absorbed, PN should not be decreased iso-calorically, especially in the initial stages.
b. Continuous enteral nutrition is the recommended mode of administration as it tends to cause less diarrhoea in patients with SBS.
c. The use of breast milk is recommended. The use of breast milk (BM) has been shown to correlate with shorter PN courses and to promote intestinal adaptation. Beneficial components of BM include high levels of nucleotides, amino acids, and immunologic and growth factors. BM also has anti-infectious properties, and glycoproteins in BM deliver iron to the intestinal epithelium, stimulate proliferation and differentiation of crypt cells, influence brush border enzyme activity, and function as scavengers to prevent free radical–mediated tissue damage.
d. Amino acid–based formulas have been associated with a shorter duration of PN-dependence when compared with standard formula and can be used if BM is not tolerated.
e. It is recommended to start oral-feeding as soon as possible. Oral feeding can be alternated with continuous enteral feeding. For example, continuous feeding might be stopped for 1 hour, and replaced by a 1-hour dose per bottle or short times of breast feeding. Solid food should be introduced at the age of 4 to 6 months, in low volumes to prevent diarrhea.
f. Animal studies have shown that administration of colostrums protein concentrate may enhance the intestinal adaptation after massive bowel resection (Nagy et al. 2004).

Neonates with SBS may have significant stool or stomal output that precludes transition to enteral feeds. Analysis of stool or stomal effluent for specific carbohydrate malabsorption (stool reducing substances and chromatography) and microscopy for fat globules will give valuable clues which will help modification of enteral formula in a rational manner. If no mechanical or infectious issues are evident, loperamide may be used to decrease stool or stomal output. Stomal re-feeding is also an effective strategy in patients with a long mucous fistula. Early stoma closure should be considered if significant fluid electrolyte imbalance occur due to high stomal loss and good length of colon is remaining.

6.1 Predictors of outcome in neonates with SBS

Eventual independence from PN support in short gut depends on various factors, including the residual length of neonatal small bowel, the health and adaptability of the remaining small bowel, presence of ileocaecal valve (ICV) and of colon. Traditionally a small bowel length of 15 cm in the presence of ICV and 40 cm in the absence of ICV have been described as minimum essential for survival in patients with short bowel syndrome. 35 cm of neonatal small bowel is associated with a 50% probability of weaning from PN (Andorsky et al. 2001).

Recent data suggests that percentage of expected small bowel for age rather than the absolute length may be a better predictor of outcomes (Wales and Christison-Lagay 2010, Diamond et al. 2010). In general, it is accepted that ileum is more adaptable than jejunum. A dilated, dysmotile gut fairs poorly than a healthy residual gut. The importance of viable colon in the survival of neonates and children with SBS is not clear with some studies showing benefit (Quiros-Tejeira et al. 2004) while the others did not (Diamond et al. 2010). The presence of colon is helpful because in patients with SBS, when undigested nutrients reach the colon it may induce changes that allow the colonic mucosa to enhance its capacity of water and electrolyte absorption as well as modifications that allow absorption of nutrients such as short- and medium-chain fatty acids. As more intact nutrients reach the colon, trophic hormones such as enteroglucagon may be stimulated, contributing to the intestinal adaptation process. Premature neonates may be at a distinct advantage with regard to intestinal adaptation (Goday 2009).

The ICV slows the transit time of intestinal contents and prevents reflux of colonic contents and bacteria into the ileum. Resection of the ICV can cause bacterial reflux into the small bowel. The ensuing bacterial overgrowth can deconjugate bile salts, reduce bile salt absorption, and impair gut function. Most studies have identified preservation of the ICV as a favourable indicator of long term adaptation although recent studies have not found the presence of intact ICV to be predictor of final outcomes (Diamond et al. 2010, Spencer et al. 2005). Citrulline is a non-structural amino acid that is primarily synthesized in the intestinal mucosa and hence reflects mucosal mass. Serum Citrulline levels correlate well with intestinal length and the ability to wean from PN. Infants with serum citrulline level persistently <15 mmol/L are usually unable to wean from PN (Fitzgibbons et al. 2009). The surgical treatment options for neonatal SBS in some centres include bowel conservation at the time of initial presentation, bowel lengthening operations and intestinal transplantation. However, recent experience suggests that the outcomes for infants and children with severe intestinal failure have improved over time and that neonates with extremely short gut, even as low as 10-20 cm of small intestine, eventually are able to be weaned off from the parenteral nutrition(Sala et al. 2010, Khalil et al. 2011).

6.2 Complications of SBS

Three specific complications are frequently associated with SBS: Intestinal Failure Associated Liver Disease (IFALD), Catheter Associated Blood Stream Infections (CABSI) and bacterial overgrowth. In addition poor growth and development will occur if adequate calories, electrolytes and micronutrients are not provided via PN.

IFALD is a common and potentially life-threatening problem for paediatric patients receiving long-term parenteral nutrition (PN). The incidence increases with the duration of TPN(Buchman 2002) and can be as high as 85% in neonates receiving TPN for prolonged periods of time. The clinical spectrum of IFALD includes hepatic steatosis, cholestasis, fibrosis, and, ultimately, progression to hepatic cirrhosis with portal hypertension and end-stage liver disease. Though the cause of IFALD is multifactorial, the single most important factor responsible is lack of enteral feeds. Other contributing factors include prematurity, reduced bile acid pool, CABSIs, chronic endotoxemia, toxic constituents in PN, excess glucose and fat in PN. Lipid emulsions derived from soybean oils have been shown to cause liver injury both in vitro and in vivo in rodent models. Preventative strategies include enteral feeding, weaning of PN, reduced dose lipid emulsions and the early recognition and treatment of sepsis. Recent studies have demonstrated the efficacy of fish-oil based lipid emulsions in the prevention and treatment of IFALD (Lilja et al. 2011, Fallon et al. 2010) and has to be incorporated in routine clinical practice. Transplantation is an option for end-stage liver disease but is associated with significant morbidity and mortality(Nehra et al. 2011).

A systematic review of observational studies concluded that Ursodeoxycholic acid may lead to short-term improvement in biochemical indices, but sample size was very small and the risk of bias very high(San Luis and Btaiche 2007). Based on the limited evidence available, ursodeoxycholic acid (10 mg/kg/dose twice or 3 times daily) may be tried in infants with IFALD who are able to tolerate some enteral intake.

CABSI can result in the loss of the central venous line, recurrent admissions to the hospital and worsen the existing liver injury. Diagnosis includes blood cultures collected from the central line. Treatment includes administration of antibiotic through the central line. In case of fulminant or resistant infection, the catheter will need to be removed. Preventative strategies include following strict protocols and aseptic precautions during insertion and management of the CVCs. A promising therapy in the prevention of CABSI is the use of ethanol locks(Wales et al. 2011). Ethanol has been demonstrated to have the ability to penetrate biofilms that form on central lines, and no bacteria or fungi have been reported to be resistant to ethanol. A recent retrospective study showed a fourfold reduction in CABSI in the cohort-administered ethanol locks (Jones et al. 2010).

Areas of disordered motility and bowel dilation in patients with SBS offer an ideal environment for abnormal bacterial propagation. The adverse effects of bacterial overgrowth include: abdominal pain, worsening motility, mucosal ulceration with bleeding, deconjugation of bile acids, and the generation of toxic byproducts such as D-lactic acid. Bacterial overgrowth can also potentiate translocation and cause septicemia. The treatment for suspected bacterial overgrowth is the administration of enteral antibiotics in a cyclical fashion. Antibiotics that are commonly used include those effective against anaerobes or Gram-negative organisms(Gutierrez et al. 2011). Systemically non absorbable antibiotics are preferred.

7. Malrotation and volvulus of the intestines in neonates

Malrotation is a serious congenital condition wherein the normal process of embryonic gut rotation is arrested or altered. The abnormal rotation usually involves both small and large bowel, within the peritoneal cavity. The most important feature is that the abnormally rotated bowel does not have a normal mesenteric attachment. The mesenteric attachment is frequently short and prone to volvulus when part of the intestine loops around the mesentery and intestines resulting in bowel obstruction and gangrene secondary to occlusion of the branches of the mesenteric artery (Figure 1a and 1b). Volvulus renders the entire bowel at risk of ischemia and necrosis. The intestinal obstruction with congenital malrotation can also result from the congenital fibrous bands (Figure 2a and 2b).

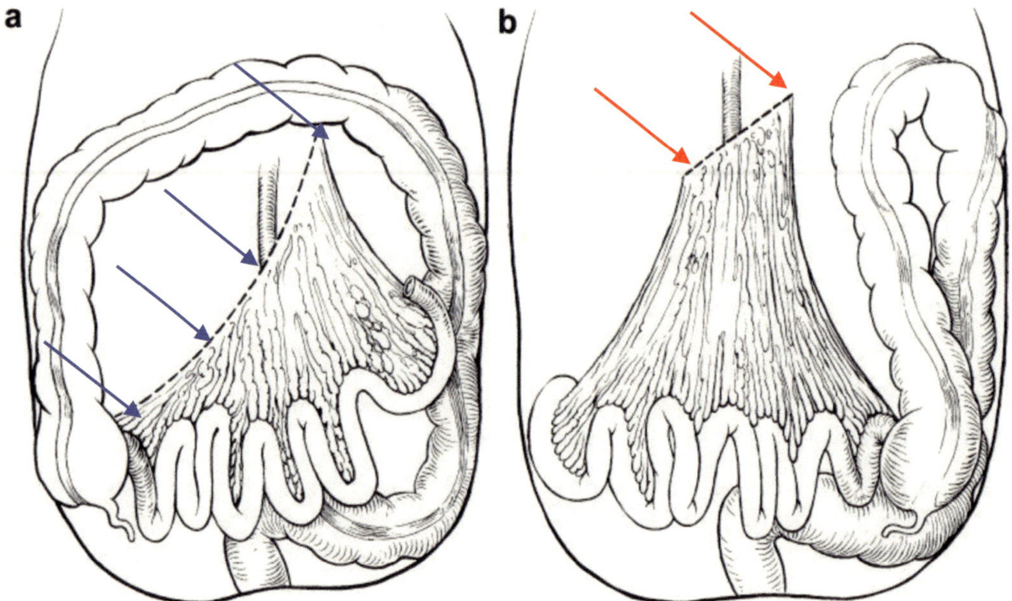

Fig. 1. a. Normal: the mesenteric root is broad, extending from the duodenojejunal junction in the left upper quadrant to the caecum in the right lower quadrant. b. Malrotation: the mesenteric root is narrow, predisposing to volvulus.

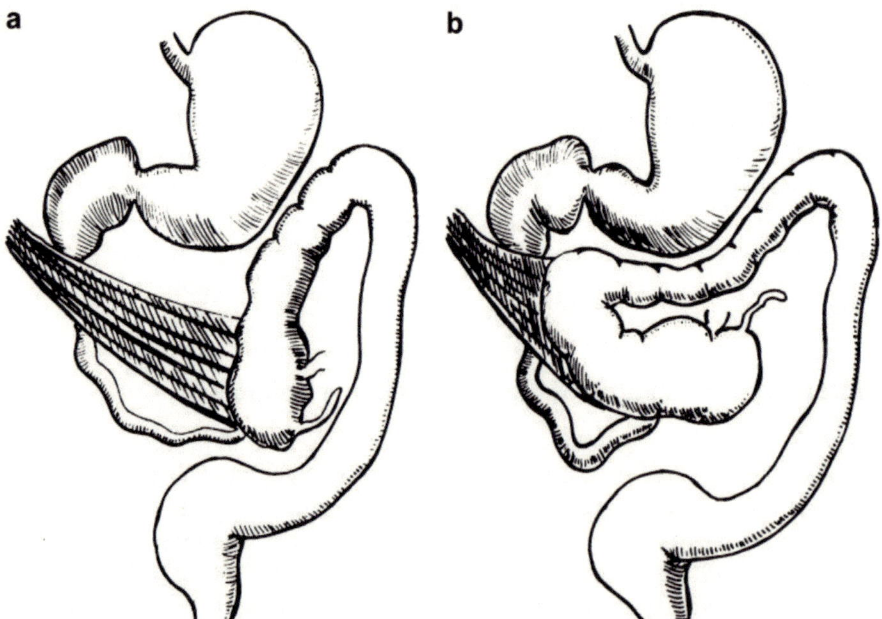

Fig. 2. Ladd's bands extend from the caecum (a) or ascending colon (b) to the right upper quadrant, passing across and variably obstructing the duodenum.

Clinical features depend on the nature and degree of obstruction (which may be intermittent) and the presence or absence of vascular compromise. Presentation can be asymptomatic but usually results in vomiting often bilious and or abdominal distension. 60–80% of patients with malrotation present in the first month of life, mostly in the first week. Bilious vomiting is an important sign of malrotation and must be promptly investigated (William 2007, Kumar 2003)). Even in the absence of bilious vomiting, malrotation/volvulus should be suspected in any neonate presenting with distended abdomen. Even though bilious aspirates can be a sign of dysmotility in extremely premature infants, persistently prolonged bilious aspirates especially lasting more than a week should raise the suspicion of malrotation. Presence of chylous fluid in the inguinal hernia sac during inguinal hernia repair should also alert the surgeons to the possibility of associated malrotation (Zarrouq 2010).

The best imaging test for the diagnosis of malrotation is an upper GI contrast study which will show an abnormal duodenum and duodeno-jejunal (DJ) flexure position (Applegate 2009). It is an emergency investigation and should not be deferred. The normal position of the DJ flexure is to the left of the spine and at the same level or higher than the duodenal bulb. In malrotation, there is no normal duodenal configuration and the proximal small bowel is in the right side of the abdomen (figure 3a and 3b).

Ultrasound and contrast enema may provide additional information but are not sufficiently accurate to exclude malrotation (Danse 2007, Chao 2000). Presence of normal lactate levels, blood pressure, urine output, blood gases do not rule out the diagnosis of intestinal gangrene secondary to malrotation/volvulus. Once a diagnosis of malrotation and or volvulus is confirmed, urgent surgical review with a view to laparotomy is indicated. Delay in the diagnosis or laparotomy may lead to ischemic necrosis of the bowel.

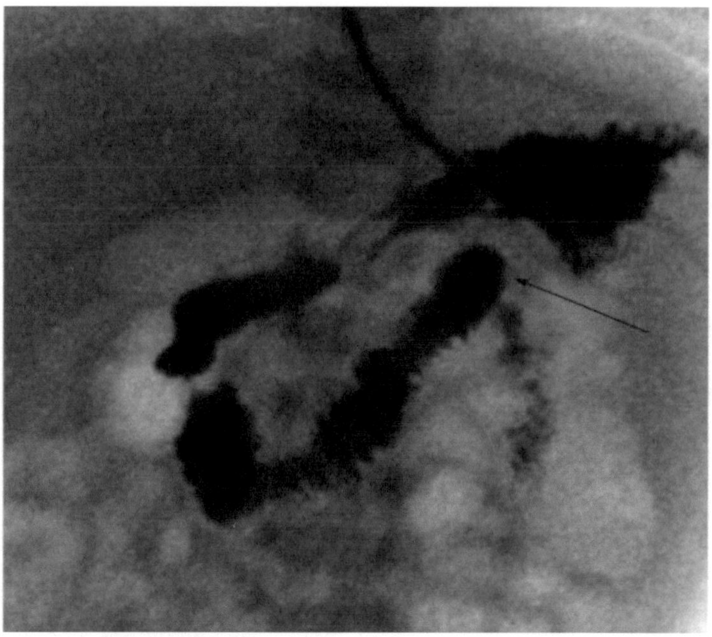

Fig. 3. a. Normal upper gastrointestinal contrast study (AP view) in a neonate with bilious vomiting. Contrast medium was introduced via a nasogastric tube. The duodeno-jejunal flexure is arrowed

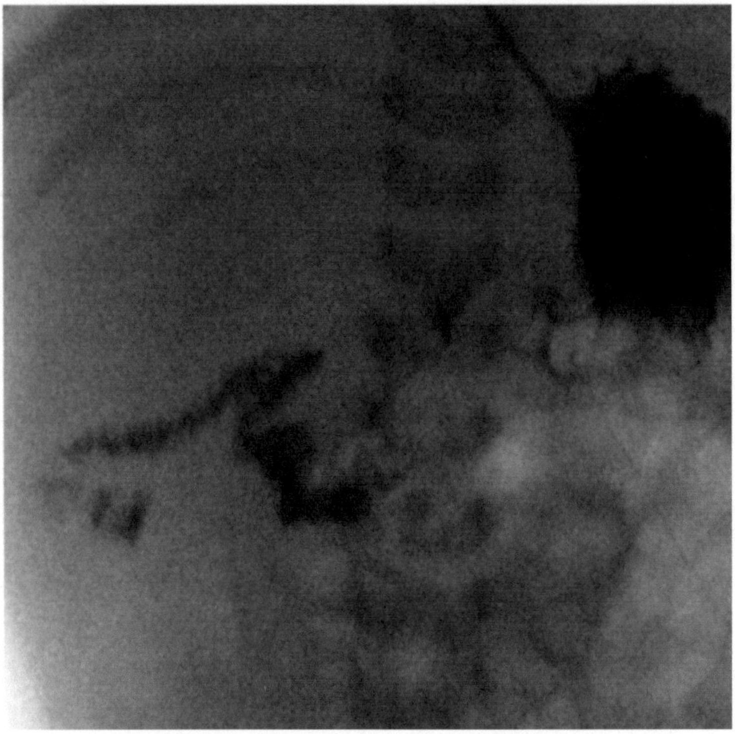

Fig. 3. b. Malrotation. There is no normal duodenal configuration and the proximal small bowel is in the right side of the abdomen.

Treatment is with the standard Ladd's procedure which involves untwisting of the volvulus, division of the Ladd's bands, broadening of the narrow base of the mesentery, division of the adhesions along the small bowel and returning the bowel in a non rotated position. Small bowel is positioned in the right abdomen and the colon in the left abdomen and appendicectomy performed (Millar 2003).

In summary, high index of suspicion, prompt investigation and early laparotomy are essential for the prevention of serious gut related morbidity and mortality secondary to malrotation and volvulus.

8. Gastroschisis

Gastroschisis is a congenital defect of the abdominal wall usually located to the right of the umbilical cord, through which abdominal organs herniate. It should be distinguished from omphalocele (or exomphalos), which results from failure of normal return of the bowel to the abdominal cavity during early fetal life. Result in herniated bowel with peritoneal covering and the umbilical cord inserted into the apex of the hernia. Distinguishing these two conditions is very important because they carry different prognoses and the temptation to combine these diseases together as 'anterior abdominal wall defects' should be avoided.

Gastroschisis occurs in up to 5 in every 10 000 live births with a sex ratio of approximately 1. Recent epidemiological surveillance data have shown a 10-20-fold increase in the overall incidence of gastroschisis in all age groups over the past two decades (Rasmussen and Frias 2008, Loane et al. 2011, Frolov et al. 2010, Clark et al. 2009).

Pathogenesis of gastroschisis is unknown, but various factors are associated with an increased risk of gastroschisis. They include young maternal age, first pregnancy, low socioeconomic status, lower pre-pregnancy body mass index (BMI), poor maternal diet, disordered family life, use of medications such as aspirin, Ibuprofen, nasal decongestants, maternal infection, smoking, alcohol cocaine, marijuana and genetic polymorphisms (Jones et al. 2009, Mac Bird et al. 2009, Rasmussen and Frias 2008).

More than 90% patients are diagnosed antenatally using ultrasound (Baird et al. 2011, Garne et al. 2010). The typical sonographic feature is multiple loops of bowel floating freely in the amniotic fluid after the time of normal embryonic return of the intestines to the abdominal cavity (10 weeks of gestation). Typically, the herniated bowel is seen to the right of the umbilical cord insertion, which is inserted normally into the anterior abdominal wall to the left of the herniated bowel. Excluding exomphalos is important in prenatal diagnosis, since exampholos is associated with aneuploidy in up to 40% of patients, and/or structural abnormalities of other organs.

Ultrasonographic assessment at regular intervals, usually every 2 weeks, is recommended after the diagnosis, to monitor foetal growth and bowel status. Development of polyhydromnios(Japaraj et al. 2003) or of progressive bowel dilatation is considered by some to indicate a poor prognosis (David et al. 2008, Payne et al. 2009) and may warrant early delivery.

Mode of delivery appears not to influence the survival or short term outcomes of gastroschisis and hence caesarean section per se for gastroschisis may not be necessary (Abdel-Latif et al. 2008). Timing of delivery is controversial with some advocating delivery before 37 weeks (Hadidi et al. 2008, Moir et al. 2004, Reigstad et al. 2011). However, since prematurity and low birth weight are associated with increased morbidities in neonates with gastroschisis, many advocate delivery at term in the absence of other obstetric complications or fetal compromise (Ergun et al. 2005, Maramreddy et al. 2009, Logghe et al. 2005).

Following delivery, adequate intravenous fluid resuscitation must be administered as there will be significant evaporative water losses from the exposed bowel. It is important to prevent intestinal distension by gastric decompression with a large bore nasogastric tube. The herniated bowel should be enclosed in a sterile plastic bag or wrapped in warm saline-soaked gauze with plastic wrap. The baby should be positioned on the right side to prevent kinking of the mesentery. The bowel needs be examined for evidence of intestinal atresia, necrosis or perforation.

Various surgical methods have been used to achieve the goal of safe reduction of the herniated viscera back into the abdominal cavity at the earliest possible time (Holland et al. 2010). Options include: (i) Complete primary reduction under general anaesthesia (ii) Complete primary reduction without the use of general anaesthesia (ward reduction) and (iii) application of preformed spring loaded silo followed by gradual reductions over few days.

Primary reduction under general anaesthesia is the traditional and commonly used approach is to reduce the viscera followed by the closure of the fascia and the skin with sutures under general anaesthesia (Owen et al. 2010). It will also enable the repair of associated anomalies such as intestinal atresia. Any significant rise in the ventilator requirements during or immediately after the surgical procedure would alert the surgeons to the possibility of abdominal compartment syndrome. In such situations, usually a silo is applied and the viscera gradually reduced over the next few days.

Primary reduction in the ward without the use of general anaesthesia practised this approach with reasonable success (Bianchi et al. 2002, Davies et al. 2005, Cauchi et al. 2006) , whereas the others have found increased complications secondary to abdominal compartment syndrome (Rao et al. 2009, Dolgin et al. 2000). The idea behind this approach is the potential for avoidance of general anaesthesia, avoidance of transfer to a surgical unit and facilitation of early enteral feeds because complete reduction has been achieved very early. This approach was pioneered in the United Kingdom, (Bianchi et al. 2002) but not adopted with enthusiasm (Owen et al. 2010). In Western Australia, this procedure has been abandoned in view of high incidence of complications(Rao et al. 2009).

Staged reduction using Silos is the preferred approach in Western Australia. Preformed spring loaded silos can be placed into the abdominal defect at the bedside to hold the herniated contents. This usually does not require general anaesthesia. Subsequently, the bowel is reduced once or twice daily into the abdominal cavity as the silo is shortened by sequential ligation. This process usually takes between one and 14 days, depending on the condition of the bowel and the infant. Definitive closure is performed once the complete reduction has been achieved. Advantages of this method are the avoidance of iatrogenic intestinal ischemia secondary to abdominal compartment syndrome. Staged reduction using preformed Silos has been found to be safe and effective in many observational studies (Owen et al. 2006, Allotey et al. 2007) and an RCT (Pastor et al. 2008) .

In situations where closure of the abdominal wall defect cannot be achieved with sutures, options are: Using umbilicus as an allograft; Prosthetic materials such as non-absorbable mesh; and biosynthetic absorbable patches such as dura or porcine small intestinal sub mucosa.

Postoperatively, it is important to watch for evidence of abdominal compartment syndrome because of the risk of iatrogenic ischemic necrosis of the bowel. Clinical features are low urine output, poor perfusion, high ventilatory requirements, need for high doses of narcotic analgesia (ischemic gut), metabolic acidosis and elevated lactate levels. Regular clinical review is extremely important and there should be low threshold for re-laparotomy. Some units use intra-gastric or urinary bladder (intra-vesical) pressures as indirect measures of intra-abdominal pressure. Values more than 20 mm Hg are thought to indicate the occurrence of this problem (Lacey et al. 1987).

A nasogastric tube should be utilized for gastric decompression in the post operative period. Feeding can commence as early as 2-3 days post operatively once haemodynamic and respiratory stability has been achieved. Early commencement of feeding can facilitate attainment of full enteral feeds soon (Sharp et al. 2000).

Gastroschisis is associated with abnormal intestinal motility and nutrient absorption, both of which gradually improve over time in most patients. Growth should be maintained with appropriate parenteral nutrition. Some infants develop short gut syndrome due to either functional dysmotility or anatomically short length of small intestines. Fish oil based lipid emulsions may be beneficial in reducing the severity or prevention of TPN associated cholestasis in such infants (Deshpande and Simmer 2011). Prokinetics such as Erythromycin have not been found to be useful for feed intolerance associated with gastroschisis (Curry et al. 2004).

Survival rate of neonates with gastroschisis is high (93-97%) (Abdel-Latif et al. 2008, Baird et al. 2011, Minutillo C 2009, Owen et al. 2010). The median time to discharge home range between 23 to 47 days (Minutillo C 2009, Baird et al. 2011), infants with short gut syndrome have very prolonged hospitalisation with the risk of complications of prolonged TPN therapy such as cholestasis and recurrent infections. Limited information available on the physical growth and neurodevelopmental outcomes suggests that treated infants have a good long term prognosis (Minutillo C 2009, Henrich et al. 2008).

In summary, the incidence of Gastroschisis has increased markedly over the past two decades. The majority of infants are diagnosed with early trimester ultrasonography. Primary reduction under general anaesthesia or gradual reduction using preformed silos is preferable and commonly used mode of reducing the contents into the abdominal cavity. A small percentage of cases develop short gut syndrome and need TPN for a protracted length of time. Survival of live born neonates with gastroschisis is very high (>93%) and limited data suggest that long term outcomes are good.

9. Neonatal hemochromatosis

Neonatal hemochromatosis(NH) is defined as severe neonatal liver disease in association with extra-hepatic iron accumulation(Whitington 2007). It is a serious disease and usually leads to death either in utero or in the early neonatal period (mortality rates 70-80%). It is the single most common cause of neonatal liver failure(Shanmugam et al. 2011).

The onset of the disease is in utero. Currently it is hypothesised to be an alloimmune process with maternal sensitization to a fetal liver antigen leading to immune injury of the fetal liver and subsequent mishandling and deposition of iron in the liver and extra hepatic tissues(Whitington 2007). Iron deposition (Siderosis) occurs in the liver and extra-hepatic tissues such as pancreas, heart, thyroid and salivary glands. Siderosis explicitly spares the reticulo-endothelial cells(Murray and Kowdley 2001).

The genetics of NH is unknown but it is not linked to the adult haemochromatosis. NH has a recurrence risk of approximately 80% within sibships of same mother but not the father, suggesting the role of a maternal alloimmune factor (Knisely et al. 2003). There are also recent reports of mitochondrial depletion syndromes presenting as NH(Hanchard et al. 2011).

Infants with NH frequently are preterm or small for gestational age. Pregnancy may be complicated by intrauterine growth retardation, oligohydramnios, placental edema, or polyhydromnios. Affected neonates develop features of liver failure with hypoalbuminemia, hypoglycemia, coagulopathy, low fibrinogen, thrombocytopenia and anaemia. If not present at birth, ascites and hyperbilirubinemia develop within a few days to weeks. Transaminase levels are generally either normal or only moderately elevated suggesting severe intrauterine hepatic damage.

NH should be suspected in any sick newborn with evidence of liver disease and in cases of late intrauterine fetal demise.

No single biochemical test is diagnostic of NH. Diagnosis is made after ruling out other causes of liver cell failure in neonates (Murray and Kowdley 2001). This includes various infectious, metabolic, storage and other disorders. In NH, Serum Ferritin levels and Transferrin saturations are raised commonly 95-100%. However, ferritin is an acute phase reactant and elevated levels are seen in many other conditions causing neonatal liver failure and hence, non-diagnostic. The hall mark of NH is extrahepatic siderosis with sparing of reticuloendothelial system. Therefore, in the face of severe coagulopathy, **Salivary gland biopsy** from the lips or cheek is a safe alternative to liver biopsy and effective way to diagnose NH(Smith et al. 2004). The histopathology of the salivary glands shows excessive iron deposition. Other conditions such as echovirus, CMV,HSV, neonatal lupus, tyrosinemia, mitochondrial diseases, rubella, parvovirus and zellweger syndrome may also cause excessive siderosis in extra hepatic organs including salivary glands and hence need to be ruled out by relevant investigations(Murray and Kowdley 2001).

On T2-weighted sequences in MRI scans, tissues with increased iron content have low signal intensity. In NH, the reticulo-endothelial system is spared so that the spleen retains a normal, higher signal intensity compared with affected tissues such as liver, heart and pancreas. Comparing the signal intensity of pancreas, heart and thyroid gland to spleen can be helpful in the diagnosis of NH (Williams et al. 2006, Tsai et al. 2009).

The differential diagnosis of neonatal liver failure include infections, perinatal asphyxia, metabolic conditions like tyrosinemia, galactosemia, Heriditary fructose intolerance, and urea cycle defects, Haemophagocytic Lymphohistiocytosis (HLH), mitochondrial disorders and Congenital disorder of glycosylation.

Supportive management involves administration of Fresh Frozen plasma, cryoprecipitate and vitamin K to normalise the coagulation abnormalities. Repeated administrations for prolonged periods are to be expected in view of ongoing liver failure.

Cocktail of antioxidants including selenium (3 microgram/kg/day orally), N acetyl-Cysteine (50-100 mg/kg/day, intravenously or orally), prostaglandin E1(0.4 microgram/kg/h, intravenously, for a maximum of two weeks), Desferoxamine 30 mg/kg/day, intravenously until the ferritin level falls to 500 ng/mL) and Vitamin E (25 IU/kg/day, orally) have been advocated (Grabhorn et al. 2006), but the results are disappointing (Heffron et al. 2007). Similar to Rand et al (2009), our suggestion is to give oral antioxidants such as vitamin E and Acetylcysteine and avoid intravenous antioxidants and chelating agents. Liver transplantation is the definitive therapy, but carries a high level of morbidity and mortality (Sundaram et al. 2003).

Recent reports have suggested the beneficial role for the treatment of NH. Double volume exchange transfusion followed by 1-3 doses of intravenous immunoglobulin (1gram/kg) has been shown to significantly improve survival without the need for liver transplantations (Rand et al. 2009). Few authors have reported beneficial outcomes with exchange transfusion alone (Timpani et al. 2007, Nicastro and Iorio 2010, Escolano-Margarit et al. 2010).

NH is the result of severe fetal liver injury that seems to result from maternal-fetal alloimmunity. Women who have had an infant affected with NH have approximately 80%

probability of recurrence in subsequent pregnancies. Recent studies have shown that weekly administration of IVIG to such pregnant mothers from 18 weeks of gestation till full term results in decreased severity of the disease and improved survival in their offsprings (Whitington and Kelly 2008, Nicholl 2010).

In summary, NH is a lethal condition and until recently, there was no effective medical therapy. Salivary gland biopsy and MRI of the abdomen are useful investigations in the diagnosis of NH. Recent studies have suggested that NH is possibly alloimmune disorder. Treatment with IVIG during pregnancy for women who had previous child with NH can prevent the occurrence and severity of NH. Exchange transfusion and IVIG may improve survival without the need for liver transplantation for neonates diagnosed with NH.

10. References

Abdel-Latif, M. E., Bolisetty, S., Abeywardana, S. & Lui, K. (2008) 'Mode of delivery and neonatal survival of infants with gastroschisis in Australia and New Zealand', *J Pediatr Surg,* 43(9), 1685-90.

Alfaleh, K., Anabrees, J., Bassler, D. and Al-Kharfi, T. (2011) 'Probiotics for prevention of necrotizing enterocolitis in preterm infants', Cochrane database of systematic reviews, (3), CD005496.

Alisi, A., Panera, N., Agostoni, C., & Nobili, V. (2011). Intrauterine growth retardation and nonalcoholic Fatty liver disease in children. *Int J Endocrinol, 2011,* 269853. doi: 10.1155/2011/269853.

Allotey, J., Davenport, M., Njere, I., Charlesworth, P., Greenough, A., Ade-Ajayi, N. & Patel, S. (2007) 'Benefit of preformed silos in the management of gastroschisis', *Pediatr Surg Int,* 23(11), 1065-9.

'American Academy of Pediatrics Committee on Nutrition: Nutritional needs of low-birth-weight infants', (1985) Pediatrics, 75(5), 976-86.

Andorsky, D. J., Lund, D. P., Lillehei, C. W., Jaksic, T., Dicanzio, J., Richardson, D. S., Collier, S. B., Lo, C. and Duggan, C. (2001) 'Nutritional and other postoperative management of neonates with short bowel syndrome correlates with clinical outcomes', J Pediatr, 139(1), 27-33.

Applegate, K. E., Anderson, J. M. & Klatte, E. C. (2006) 'Intestinal malrotation in children: a problem-solving approach to the upper gastrointestinal series', *Radiographics,* 26(5), 1485-500.

Applegate, K.E. (2009) 'Evidence-based diagnosis of malrotation and volvulus', *Pediatr Radiol', 39 Suppl,* 2:S161-3.

Babson, S. G. and Benda, G. I. (1976) 'Growth graphs for the clinical assessment of infants of varying gestational age', J Pediatr, 89(5), 814-20.

Baird, R., Eeson, G., Safavi, A., Puligandla, P., Laberge, J. M. & Skarsgard, E. D. (2011) 'Institutional practice and outcome variation in the management of congenital diaphragmatic hernia and gastroschisis in Canada: a report from the Canadian Pediatric Surgery Network', *J Pediatr Surg,* 46(5), 801-7.

Barker, D. J. (2004). The developmental origins of well-being. *Philos Trans R Soc Lond B Biol Sci, 359*(1449), 1359-1366. doi: 10.1098/rstb.2004.1518.

Barrington, K. J. (2011) 'Review: probiotics prevented necrotising enterocolitis and reduced mortality in preterm neonates', Archives of disease in childhood. Education and practice edition.

Beeby, P. J., Bhutap, T. and Taylor, L. K. (1996) 'New South Wales population-based birthweight percentile charts', J Paediatr Child Health, 32(6), 512-8.

Berg, A., Kramer, U., Link, E., Bollrath, C., Heinrich, J., Brockow, I., Koletzko, S., Grubl, A., Filipiak-Pittroff, B., Wichmann, H. E., Bauer, C. P., Reinhardt, D. and Berdel, D. (2010) 'Impact of early feeding on childhood eczema: development after nutritional intervention compared with the natural course - the GINIplus study up to the age of 6 years', Clinical and experimental allergy : journal of the British Society for Allergy and Clinical Immunology, 40(4), 627-36.

Bernstein, I. M., Horbar, J. D., Badger, G. J., Ohlsson, A., & Golan, A. (2000). Morbidity and mortality among very-low-birth-weight neonates with intrauterine growth restriction. The Vermont Oxford Network. *Am J Obstet Gynecol, 182*(1 Pt 1), 198-206.

Berrington, J. E., Hearn, R. I., Bythell, M., Wright, C. and Embleton, N. D. (2011) 'Deaths in Preterm Infants: Changing Pathology Over 2 Decades', The Journal of pediatrics.

Berseth, C. L., Bisquera, J. A. and Paje, V. U. (2003) 'Prolonging small feeding volumes early in life decreases the incidence of necrotizing enterocolitis in very low birth weight infants', Pediatrics, 111(3), 529-34.

Bertino, E., Coscia, A., Mombro, M., Boni, L., Rossetti, G., Fabris, C., Spada, E. and Milani, S. (2006) 'Postnatal weight increase and growth velocity of very low birthweight infants', Arch Dis Child Fetal Neonatal Ed, 91(5), F349-56.

Bertino, E., Milani, S., Fabris, C. and De Curtis, M. (2007) 'Neonatal anthropometric charts: what they are, what they are not', Arch Dis Child Fetal Neonatal Ed, 92(1), F7-F10.

Bhide, A. (2011). Fetal growth restriction and developmental delay: current understanding and future possibilities. *Ultrasound Obstet Gynecol, 38*(3), 243-245. doi: 10.1002/uog.10055.

Bianchi, A., Dickson, A. P. & Alizai, N. K. (2002) 'Elective delayed midgut reduction-No anesthesia for gastroschisis: Selection and conversion criteria', *J Pediatr Surg,* 37(9), 1334-6.

Breeze, A. C., & Lees, C. C. (2007). Prediction and perinatal outcomes of fetal growth restriction. *Semin Fetal Neonatal Med, 12*(5), 383-397. doi: 10.1016/j.siny.2007.07.002.

Buchman, A. (2002) 'Total parenteral nutrition-associated liver disease', JPEN J Parenter Enteral Nutr, 26(5 Suppl), S43-8.

Casey, P. H., Whiteside-Mansell, L., Barrett, K., Bradley, R. H. and Gargus, R. (2006) 'Impact of prenatal and/or postnatal growth problems in low birth weight preterm infants on school-age outcomes: an 8-year longitudinal evaluation', Pediatrics, 118(3), 1078-86.

Cauchi, J., Parikh, D. H., Samuel, M. & Gornall, P. (2006) 'Does gastroschisis reduction require general anesthesia? A comparative analysis', *J Pediatr Surg,* 41(7), 1294-7.

Chao, H. C., Kong, M. S, Chen, J. Y, Lin, S. J. & Lin, J. N. (2000) 'Sonographic features related to volvulus in neonatal intestinal malrotation', *J Ultrasound Med,* 19(6), 371-6.

Chauhan, S. P., Hendrix, N. W., Magann, E. F., Morrison, J. C., Scardo, J. A. and Berghella, V. (2005) 'A review of sonographic estimate of fetal weight: vagaries of accuracy', J Matern Fetal Neonatal Med, 18(4), 211-20.

Clark, R. H., Walker, M. W. & Gauderer, M. W. (2009) 'Prevalence of gastroschisis and associated hospital time continue to rise in neonates who are admitted for intensive care', *J Pediatr Surg,* 44(6), 1108-12.

Claud, E. C. and Walker, W. A. (2001) 'Hypothesis: inappropriate colonization of the premature intestine can cause neonatal necrotizing enterocolitis', The FASEB journal: official publication of the Federation of American Societies for Experimental Biology, 15(8), 1398-403.

Cleal, J. K., Poore, K. R., Boullin, J. P., Khan, O., Chau, R., Hambidge, O., et al. (2007). Mismatched pre- and postnatal nutrition leads to cardiovascular dysfunction and altered renal function in adulthood. *Proc Natl Acad Sci U S A, 104*(22), 9529-9533. doi: 0610373104 [pii] 10.1073/pnas.0610373104 [doi].

Cooke, R. J., Griffin, I. J. and McCormick, K. (2010) 'Adiposity is not altered in preterm infants fed with a nutrient-enriched formula after hospital discharge', Pediatric research, 67(6), 660-4.

Curry, J. I., Lander, A. D. & Stringer, M. D. (2004) 'A multicenter, randomized, double-blind, placebo-controlled trial of the prokinetic agent erythromycin in the postoperative recovery of infants with gastroschisis', *J Pediatr Surg,* 39(4), 565-9.

Damodaram, M., Story, L., Kulinskaya, E., Rutherford, M., & Kumar, S. (2011). Early adverse perinatal complications in preterm growth-restricted fetuses. *Aust N Z J Obstet Gynaecol, 51*(3), 204-209. doi: 10.1111/j.1479-82 8X.2011.01299.x.

Danse, E. M., Kartheuser, A., Paterson, H. M. & Laterre, P. F. (2009) 'Color Doppler sonography of small bowel wall changes in 21 consecutive cases of acute mesenteric ischemia,' *JBR-BTR,* 92(4), 202-6.

Darlow, B. A. and Graham, P. J. (2007) 'Vitamin A supplementation to prevent mortality and short and long-term morbidity in very low birthweight infants', Cochrane database of systematic reviews, (4), CD000501.

David, A. L., Tan, A. & Curry, J. (2008) 'Gastroschisis: sonographic diagnosis, associations, management and outcome', *Prenat Diagn,* 28(7), 633-44.

Davies, M. W., Kimble, R. M. & Cartwright, D. W. (2005) 'Gastroschisis: ward reduction compared with traditional reduction under general anesthesia', *J Pediatr Surg,* 40(3), 523-7.

De Curtis, M., & Rigo, J. (2004). Extrauterine growth restriction in very-low-birthweight infants. *Acta Paediatr, 93,* 1563-1568.

Deshpande, G. & Simmer, K. (2011) 'Lipids for parenteral nutrition in neonates', *Curr Opin Clin Nutr Metab Care,* 14(2), 145-50.

Deshpande, G. and Simmer, K. (2011) 'Lipids for parenteral nutrition in neonates', Current opinion in clinical nutrition and metabolic care, 14(2), 145-50.

Deshpande, G. C., Rao, S. C., Keil, A. D. and Patole, S. K. (2011) 'Evidence-based guidelines for use of probiotics in preterm neonates', BMC medicine, 9, 92.

Deshpande, G., Rao, S., Patole, S. and Bulsara, M. (2010) 'Updated meta-analysis of probiotics for preventing necrotizing enterocolitis in preterm neonates', Pediatrics, 125(5), 921-30.

Deshpande, G., Rao, S., Patole, S. and Bulsara, M. (2010) 'Updated meta-analysis of probiotics for preventing necrotizing enterocolitis in preterm neonates', Pediatrics, 125(5), 921-30.

Diamond, I. R., Struijs, M. C., de Silva, N. T. and Wales, P. W. (2010) 'Does the colon play a role in intestinal adaptation in infants with short bowel syndrome? A multiple variable analysis', J Pediatr Surg, 45(5), 975-9.

Diekmann, M., Genzel-Boroviczeny, O., Zoppelli, L. and von Poblotzki, M. (2005) 'Postnatal growth curves for extremely low birth weight infants with early enteral nutrition', Eur J Pediatr, 164(12), 714-23.

Dinerstein, A., Nieto, R. M., Solana, C. L., Perez, G. P., Otheguy, L. E. and Larguia, A. M. (2006) 'Early and aggressive nutritional strategy (parenteral and enteral) decreases postnatal growth failure in very low birth weight infants', Journal of perinatology : official journal of the California Perinatal Association, 26(7), 436-42.

Dolgin, S. E., Midulla, P. & Shlasko, E. (2000) 'Unsatisfactory experience with 'minimal intervention management' for gastroschisis', *J Pediatr Surg,* 35(10), 1437-9.

Dudley, N. J. (2005) 'A systematic review of the ultrasound estimation of fetal weight', Ultrasound Obstet Gynecol, 25(1), 80-9.

Dusick, A. M., Poindexter, B. B., Ehrenkranz, R. A. and Lemons, J. A. (2003) 'Growth failure in the preterm infant: can we catch up?', Seminars in perinatology, 27(4), 302-10.

Ehrenkranz, R. A., Dusick, A. M., Vohr, B. R., Wright, L. L., Wrage, L. A. and Poole, W. K. (2006) 'Growth in the neonatal intensive care unit influences neurodevelopmental and growth outcomes of extremely low birth weight infants', Pediatrics, 117(4), 1253-61.

Ehrenkranz, R. A., Dusick, A. M., Vohr, B. R., Wright, L. L., Wrage, L. A. and Poole, W. K. (2006) 'Growth in the neonatal intensive care unit influences neurodevelopmental and growth outcomes of extremely low birth weight infants', Pediatrics, 117(4), 1253-61.

Ekelund, U., Ong, K., Linne, Y., Neovius, M., Brage, S., Dunger, D. B., Wareham, N. J. and Rossner, S. (2006) 'Upward weight percentile crossing in infancy and early childhood independently predicts fat mass in young adults: the Stockholm Weight Development Study (SWEDES)', Am J Clin Nutr, 83(2), 324-30.

Ergun, O., Barksdale, E., Ergun, F. S., Prosen, T., Qureshi, F. G., Reblock, K. R., Ford, H. and Hackam, D. J. (2005) 'The timing of delivery of infants with gastroschisis influences outcome', *J Pediatr Surg,* 40(2), 424-8.

Escolano-Margarit, M. V., Miras-Baldo, M. J., Parrilla-Roure, M., Rivera-Cuello, M. and Narbona-Lopez, E. (2010) 'Exchange transfusion as a possible therapy for neonatal hemochromatosis', Journal of pediatric gastroenterology and nutrition, 50(5), 566-8.

Euser, A. M., Finken, M. J., Keijzer-Veen, M. G., Hille, E. T., Wit, J. M. and Dekker, F. W. (2005) 'Associations between prenatal and infancy weight gain and BMI, fat mass, and fat distribution in young adulthood: a prospective cohort study in males and females born very preterm', Am J Clin Nutr, 81(2), 480-7.

Fallon, E. M., Le, H. D. and Puder, M. (2010) 'Prevention of parenteral nutrition-associated liver disease: role of omega-3 fish oil', Curr Opin Organ Transplant, 15(3), 334-40.

Fanaro, S. (2010) 'Which is the ideal target for preterm growth?', Minerva pediatrica, 62(3 Suppl 1), 77-82.

Fenton, T. R. (2003) 'A new growth chart for preterm babies: Babson and Benda's chart updated with recent data and a new format', BMC Pediatr, 3, 13.

Figueras, F., & Gardosi, J. (2011). Intrauterine growth restriction: new concepts in antenatal surveillance, diagnosis, and management. *Am J Obstet Gynecol, 204*(4), 288-300. doi: 10.1016/j.ajog.2010.08.055.

Finken, M. J., Keijzer-Veen, M. G., Dekker, F. W., Frolich, M., Hille, E. T., Romijn, J. A. and Wit, J. M. (2006) 'Preterm birth and later insulin resistance: effects of birth weight and postnatal growth in a population based longitudinal study from birth into adult life', Diabetologia, 49(3), 478-85.

'http://www.intergrowth21.org.uk/', (Accessed 18 September, 2011) [online], available: [accessed 18 September, 2011].

Fitzgibbons, S., Ching, Y. A., Valim, C., Zhou, J., Iglesias, J., Duggan, C. and Jaksic, T. (2009) 'Relationship between serum citrulline levels and progression to parenteral nutrition independence in children with short bowel syndrome', J Pediatr Surg, 44(5), 928-32.

Frolov, P., Alali, J. & Klein, M. D. (2010) 'Clinical risk factors for gastroschisis and omphalocele in humans: a review of the literature', *Pediatr Surg Int.*

Garne, E., Dolk, H., Loane, M. & Boyd, P. A. (2010) 'EUROCAT website data on prenatal detection rates of congenital anomalies', *J Med Screen,* 17(2), 97-8.

Goday, P. S. (2009) 'Short bowel syndrome: how short is too short?', Clin Perinatol, 36(1), 101-10.

Goldenberg, R. L., Cutter, G. R., Hoffman, H. J., Foster, J. M., Nelson, K. G., & Hauth, J. C. (1989). Intrauterine growth retardation: standards for diagnosis. *Am J Obstet Gynecol, 161*(2), 271-277.

Goulet, O. and Ruemmele, F. (2006) 'Causes and management of intestinal failure in children', Gastroenterology, 130(2 Suppl 1), S16-28.

Grabhorn, E., Richter, A., Burdelski, M., Rogiers, X. and Ganschow, R. (2006) 'Neonatal hemochromatosis: long-term experience with favorable outcome', Pediatrics, 118(5), 2060-5.

Gutierrez, I. M., Kang, K. H. and Jaksic, T. (2011) 'Neonatal short bowel syndrome', Semin Fetal Neonatal Med, 16(3), 157-63.

Hadidi, A., Subotic, U., Goeppl, M. & Waag, K. L. (2008) 'Early elective cesarean delivery before 36 weeks vs late spontaneous delivery in infants with gastroschisis', *J Pediatr Surg,* 43(7), 1342-6.

Hanchard, N. A., Shchelochkov, O. A., Roy, A., Wiszniewska, J., Wang, J., Popek, E. J., Karpen, S., Wong, L. J. and Scaglia, F. (2011) 'Deoxyguanosine kinase deficiency presenting as neonatal hemochromatosis', Mol Genet Metab, 103(3), 262-7.

Hartmann, B. T., Pang, W. W., Keil, A. D., Hartmann, P. E. and Simmer, K. (2007) 'Best practice guidelines for the operation of a donor human milk bank in an Australian NICU', Early human development, 83(10), 667-73.

Hay, W. W., Jr. (2008). Strategies for feeding the preterm infant. *Neonatology, 94*(4), 245-254. doi: 000151643 [pii] 10.1159/000151643 [doi].

Heffron, T., Pillen, T., Welch, D., Asolati, M., Smallwood, G., Hagedorn, P., Fasola, C., Solis, D., Rodrigues, J., DePaolo, J., Spivey, J., Martinez, E., Henry, S. and Romero, R. (2007) 'Medical and surgical treatment of neonatal hemochromatosis: single center experience', Pediatric transplantation, 11(4), 374-8.

Henrich, K., Huemmer, H. P., Reingruber, B. & Weber, P. G. (2008) 'Gastroschisis and omphalocele: treatments and long-term outcomes', *Pediatr Surg Int,* 24(2), 167-73.

Holland, A. J., Walker, K. & Badawi, N. (2010) 'Gastroschisis: an update', *Pediatr Surg Int,* 26(9), 871-8.

Japaraj, R. P., Hockey, R. & Chan, F. Y. (2003) 'Gastroschisis: can prenatal sonography predict neonatal outcome?', *Ultrasound Obstet Gynecol,* 21(4), 329-33.

Johnsen, S. L., Rasmussen, S., Wilsgaard, T., Sollien, R. and Kiserud, T. (2006) 'Longitudinal reference ranges for estimated fetal weight', Acta Obstet Gynecol Scand, 85(3), 286-97.

Jones, B. A., Hull, M. A., Richardson, D. S., Zurakowski, D., Gura, K., Fitzgibbons, S. C., Duro, D., Lo, C. W., Duggan, C. and Jaksic, T. (2010) 'Efficacy of ethanol locks in reducing central venous catheter infections in pediatric patients with intestinal failure', J Pediatr Surg, 45(6), 1287-93.

Jones, K. L., Benirschke, K. & Chambers, C. D. (2009) 'Gastroschisis: etiology and developmental pathogenesis', *Clin Genet,* 75(4), 322-5.

Karna, P., Brooks, K., Muttineni, J. and Karmaus, W. (2005) 'Anthropometric measurements for neonates, 23 to 29 weeks gestation, in the 1990s', Paediatr Perinat Epidemiol, 19(3), 215-26.

Kennedy, K. A., Tyson, J. E. and Chamnanvanakij, S. (2000) 'Rapid versus slow rate of advancement of feedings for promoting growth and preventing necrotizing enterocolitis in parenterally fed low-birth-weight infants', Cochrane database of systematic reviews, (2), CD001241.

Khalil, B. A., Ba'ath, M. E., Aziz, A., Forsythe, L., Gozzini, S., Murphy, F., Carlson, G., Bianchi, A. and Morabito, A. (2011) 'Intestinal Rehabilitation And Bowel Reconstructive Surgery: Improved Outcomes In Children With Short Bowel Syndrome', Journal of pediatric gastroenterology and nutrition.

Knisely, A. S., Mieli-Vergani, G. and Whitington, P. F. (2003) 'Neonatal hemochromatosis', Gastroenterology clinics of North America, 32(3), 877-89, vi-vii.

Kocoshis, S. A. (2010) 'Medical management of pediatric intestinal failure', Semin Pediatr Surg, 19(1), 20-6.

Koletzko, B., Krohn, K., Goulet, O. and Shamir, R. (2008) Paediatric Parenteral nutrition. A practical reference guide, KARGER.

Kramer, M. S., Platt, R. W., Wen, S. W., Joseph, K. S., Allen, A., Abrahamowicz, M., Blondel, B. and Breart, G. (2001) 'A new and improved population-based Canadian reference for birth weight for gestational age', Pediatrics, 108(2), E35.

Kumar, N., Curry, J. I. (2008) 'Bile-stained vomiting in the infant: green is not good!', *Arch Dis Child Educ Pract Ed,* 93(3):84-6.

Lacey, S. R., Bruce, J., Brooks, S. P., Griswald, J., Ferguson, W., Allen, J. E., Jewett, T. C., Jr., Karp, M. P. & Cooney, D. R. (1987) 'The relative merits of various methods of indirect measurement of intraabdominal pressure as a guide to closure of abdominal wall defects', *Journal of pediatric surgery,* 22(12), 1207-11.

Latal-Hajnal, B., von Siebenthal, K., Kovari, H., Bucher, H. U. and Largo, R. H. (2003) 'Postnatal growth in VLBW infants: significant association with neurodevelopmental outcome', The Journal of pediatrics, 143(2), 163-70.

Latal-Hajnal, B., von Siebenthal, K., Kovari, H., Bucher, H. U. and Largo, R. H. (2003) 'Postnatal growth in VLBW infants: significant association with neurodevelopmental outcome', The Journal of pediatrics, 143(2), 163-70.

Levene, M., Tudehope, D., & Thearle, M. (2000). *Neonatal Medicine* (3 ed.). Oxford, UK: Blackwell Publishing Company.

Lilja, H. E., Finkel, Y., Paulsson, M. and Lucas, S. (2011) 'Prevention and reversal of intestinal failure-associated liver disease in premature infants with short bowel syndrome using intravenous fish oil in combination with omega-6/9 lipid emulsions', J Pediatr Surg, 46(7), 1361-7.

Loane, M., Dolk, H., Kelly, A., Teljeur, C., Greenlees, R. & Densem, J. (2011) 'Paper 4: EUROCAT statistical monitoring: identification and investigation of ten year trends of congenital anomalies in Europe', *Birth Defects Res A Clin Mol Teratol,* 91 Suppl 1, S31-43.

Logghe, H. L., Mason, G. C., Thornton, J. G. & Stringer, M. D. (2005) 'A randomized controlled trial of elective preterm delivery of fetuses with gastroschisis', *J Pediatr Surg,* 40(11), 1726-31.

Lubchenco, L. O., Hansman, C., Dressler, M., & Boyd, E. (1963). Intrauterine growth as estimated from liveborn birth-weight data at 24 to 42 weeks of gestation. *Pediatrics, 32,* 793-800.

Mac Bird, T., Robbins, J. M., Druschel, C., Cleves, M. A., Yang, S. & Hobbs, C. A. (2009) 'Demographic and environmental risk factors for gastroschisis and omphalocele in the National Birth Defects Prevention Study', *J Pediatr Surg,* 44(8), 1546-51.

Makrides, M., Gibson, R. A., McPhee, A. J., Collins, C. T., Davis, P. G., Doyle, L. W., Simmer, K., Colditz, P. B., Morris, S., Smithers, L. G., Willson, K. and Ryan, P. (2009) 'Neurodevelopmental outcomes of preterm infants fed high-dose docosahexaenoic acid: a randomized controlled trial', JAMA : the journal of the American Medical Association, 301(2), 175-82.

Maramreddy, H., Fisher, J., Slim, M., Lagamma, E. F. & Parvez, B. (2009) 'Delivery of gastroschisis patients before 37 weeks of gestation is associated with increased morbidities', *J Pediatr Surg,* 44(7), 1360-6.

Millar, A. J., Rode, H. & Cywes, S. (2003) 'Malrotation and volvulus in infancy and childhood', *Semin Pediatr Surg,* 12(4), 229-36.

Millar, M., Wilks, M. and Costeloe, K. (2003) 'Probiotics for preterm infants?', Archives of disease in childhood. Fetal and neonatal edition, 88(5), F354-8.

Minutillo C, P. S., McMichael J, Dickinson JE & Rao S. C. (2009) 'Neurodevelopmental outcomes of infants with gastroschisis in Western Australia: A retrospective study, translated by Darwin, NT, Australia', *Journal of Paediatrics and Child Health,* A171.

Moir, C. R., Ramsey, P. S., Ogburn, P. L., Johnson, R. V. & Ramin, K. D. (2004) 'A prospective trial of elective preterm delivery for fetal gastroschisis', *Am J Perinatol,* 21(5), 289-94.

Morgan, J. A., Young, L. and McGuire, W. (2011) 'Pathogenesis and prevention of necrotizing enterocolitis', Current opinion in infectious diseases, 24(3), 183-9.

Morrison, J. L., Duffield, J. A., Muhlhausler, B. S., Gentili, S. and McMillen, I. C. (2010) 'Fetal growth restriction, catch-up growth and the early origins of insulin resistance and visceral obesity', Pediatric nephrology, 25(4), 669-77.

Murray, K. F. and Kowdley, K. V. (2001) 'Neonatal hemochromatosis', Pediatrics, 108(4), 960-4.

Nagy, E. S., Paris, M. C., Taylor, R. G., Fuller, P. J., Sourial, M., Justice, F. and Bines, J. E. (2004) 'Colostrum protein concentrate enhances intestinal adaptation after massive small bowel resection in juvenile pigs', J Pediatr Gastroenterol Nutr, 39(5), 487-92.

Nehra, D., Fallon, E. M. and Puder, M. (2011) 'The Prevention and Treatment of Intestinal Failure-associated Liver Disease in Neonates and Children', Surg Clin North Am, 91(3), 543-63.

Neu, J. and Shuster, J. (2010) 'Nonadministration of routine probiotics unethical--really?', Pediatrics, 126(3), e740-1; author reply e743-5.

Nicastro, E. and Iorio, R. (2010) 'Neonatal hemochromatosis and exchange transfusion: treating the disorder as an alloimmune disease', Journal of pediatric gastroenterology and nutrition, 50(5), 471-2.

Nicholl, M. C. (2010) 'Successful pregnancy outcome with the use of antenatal high-dose intravenous immunoglobulin following previous neonatal death associated with neonatal haemochromatosis', The Australian & New Zealand journal of obstetrics & gynaecology, 50(4), 403-5.

Niklasson, A., Ericson, A., Fryer, J. G., Karlberg, J., Lawrence, C. and Karlberg, P. (1991) 'An update of the Swedish reference standards for weight, length and head circumference at birth for given gestational age (1977-1981)', Acta Paediatr Scand, 80(8-9), 756-62.

'Nutrient needs and feeding of premature infants. Nutrition Committee, Canadian Paediatric Society', (1995) CMAJ, 152(11), 1765-85.

Oh, W., Poindexter, B. B., Perritt, R., Lemons, J. A., Bauer, C. R., Ehrenkranz, R. A., Stoll, B. J., Poole, K. and Wright, L. L. (2005) 'Association between fluid intake and weight loss during the first ten days of life and risk of bronchopulmonary dysplasia in extremely low birth weight infants', J Pediatr, 147(6), 786-90.

O'Keefe, S. J., Buchman, A. L., Fishbein, T. M., Jeejeebhoy, K. N., Jeppesen, P. B. and Shaffer, J. (2006) 'Short bowel syndrome and intestinal failure: consensus definitions and overview', Clinical gastroenterology and hepatology : the official clinical practice journal of the American Gastroenterological Association, 4(1), 6-10.

Olieman, J. F., Penning, C., Ijsselstijn, H., Escher, J. C., Joosten, K. F., Hulst, J. M. and Tibboel, D. (2010) 'Enteral nutrition in children with short-bowel syndrome: current evidence and recommendations for the clinician', J Am Diet Assoc, 110(3), 420-6.

Olsen, I. E., Groveman, S. A., Lawson, M. L., Clark, R. H., & Zemel, B. S. (2010). New intrauterine growth curves based on United States data. *Pediatrics, 125*(2), e214-224. doi: 10.1542/peds.2009-0913.

Ong, K. K. (2007) 'Catch-up growth in small for gestational age babies: good or bad?', Current opinion in endocrinology, diabetes, and obesity, 14(1), 30-4.

Owen, A., Marven, S., Jackson, L., Antao, B., Roberts, J., Walker, J. & Shawis, R. (2006) 'Experience of bedside preformed silo staged reduction and closure for gastroschisis', *J Pediatr Surg,* 41(11), 1830-5.

Owen, A., Marven, S., Johnson, P., Kurinczuk, J., Spark, P., Draper, E. S., Brocklehurst, P. & Knight, M. (2010) 'Gastroschisis: a national cohort study to describe contemporary surgical strategies and outcomes', *J Pediatr Surg,* 45(9), 1808-16.

Ozanne, S. E., & Hales, C. N. (2004). Lifespan: catch-up growth and obesity in male mice. *Nature, 427*(6973), 411-412.

Pastor, A. C., Phillips, J. D., Fenton, S. J., Meyers, R. L., Lamm, A. W., Raval, M. V., Lehman, E., Karp, T. B., Wales, P. W. & Langer, J. C. (2008) 'Routine use of a SILASTIC spring-loaded silo for infants with gastroschisis: a multicenter randomized controlled trial', *J Pediatr Surg,* 43(10), 1807-12.

Payne, N. R., Pfleghaar, K., Assel, B., Johnson, A. & Rich, R. H. (2009) 'Predicting the outcome of newborns with gastroschisis', *J Pediatr Surg,* 44(5), 918-23.

Poindexter, B. B., Langer, J. C., Dusick, A. M. and Ehrenkranz, R. A. (2006) 'Early provision of parenteral amino acids in extremely low birth weight infants: relation to growth and neurodevelopmental outcome', The Journal of pediatrics, 148(3), 300-305.

Quigley, M. A., Henderson, G., Anthony, M. Y. and McGuire, W. (2007) 'Formula milk versus donor breast milk for feeding preterm or low birth weight infants', Cochrane database of systematic reviews, (4), CD002971.

Quiros-Tejeira, R. E., Ament, M. E., Reyen, L., Herzog, F., Merjanian, M., Olivares-Serrano, N. and Vargas, J. H. (2004) 'Long-term parenteral nutritional support and intestinal adaptation in children with short bowel syndrome: a 25-year experience', J Pediatr, 145(2), 157-63.

Rand, E. B., Karpen, S. J., Kelly, S., Mack, C. L., Malatack, J. J., Sokol, R. J. and Whitington, P. F. (2009) 'Treatment of neonatal hemochromatosis with exchange transfusion and intravenous immunoglobulin', The Journal of pediatrics, 155(4), 566-71.

Rao, S. C., Pirie, S., Minutillo, C., Gollow, I., Dickinson, J. E. & Jacoby, P. (2009) 'Ward reduction of gastroschisis in a single stage without general anaesthesia may increase the risk of short-term morbidities: Results of a retrospective audit', *J Paediatr Child Health.*

Rasmussen, S. A. & Frias, J. L. (2008) 'Non-genetic risk factors for gastroschisis', *Am J Med Genet C Semin Med Genet,* 148C(3), 199-212.

Reigstad, I., Reigstad, H., Kiserud, T. & Berstad, T. (2011) 'Preterm elective caesarean section and early enteral feeding in gastroschisis', *Acta Paediatr,* 100(1), 71-4.

Resnik, R. (2002). Intrauterine growth restriction. *Obstet Gynecol, 99*(3), 490-496.

Ronnestad, A., Abrahamsen, T. G., Medbo, S., Reigstad, H., Lossius, K., Kaaresen, P. I., Egeland, T., Engelund, I. E., Irgens, L. M. and Markestad, T. (2005) 'Late-onset septicemia in a Norwegian national cohort of extremely premature infants receiving very early full human milk feeding', Pediatrics, 115(3), e269-76.

Sala, D., Chomto, S. and Hill, S. (2010) 'Long-term outcomes of short bowel syndrome requiring long-term/home intravenous nutrition compared in children with gastroschisis and those with volvulus', Transplant Proc, 42(1), 5-8.

San Luis, V. A. and Btaiche, I. F. (2007) 'Ursodiol in patients with parenteral nutrition-associated cholestasis', Ann Pharmacother, 41(11), 1867-72.

Schanler, R. J. (2001) 'The use of human milk for premature infants', Pediatric clinics of North America, 48(1), 207-19.

Schulzke, S. M., Deshpande, G. C. and Patole, S. K. (2007) 'Neurodevelopmental outcomes of very low-birth-weight infants with necrotizing enterocolitis: a systematic review of observational studies', Archives of pediatrics & adolescent medicine, 161(6), 583-90.

Schulzke, S. M., Patole, S. K. and Simmer, K. (2011) 'Longchain polyunsaturated fatty acid supplementation in preterm infants', Cochrane database of systematic reviews, (2), CD000375.

Shah, P. S., Wong, K. Y., Merko, S., Bishara, R., Dunn, M., Asztalos, E. and Darling, P. B. (2006) 'Postnatal growth failure in preterm infants: ascertainment and relation to long-term outcome', J Perinat Med, 34(6), 484-9.

Shanmugam, N. P., Bansal, S., Greenough, A., Verma, A. and Dhawan, A. (2011) 'Neonatal liver failure: aetiologies and management--state of the art', Eur J Pediatr, 170(5), 573-81.

Sharp, M., Bulsara, M., Gollow, I. & Pemberton, P. (2000) 'Gastroschisis: early enteral feeds may improve outcome', *J Paediatr Child Health,* 36(5), 472-6.

Sices, L., Wilson-Costello, D., Minich, N., Friedman, H. and Hack, M. (2007) 'Postdischarge growth failure among extremely low birth weight infants: Correlates and consequences', Paediatr Child Health, 12(1), 22-8.

Simmer, K. and Rao, S. C. (2005) 'Early introduction of lipids to parenterally-fed preterm infants', Cochrane database of systematic reviews, (2), CD005256.

Singhal, A., Cole, T. J., Fewtrell, M., Kennedy, K., Stephenson, T., Elias-Jones, A. and Lucas, A. (2007) 'Promotion of faster weight gain in infants born small for gestational age: is there an adverse effect on later blood pressure?', Circulation, 115(2), 213-20.

Smith, S. R., Shneider, B. L., Magid, M., Martin, G. and Rothschild, M. (2004) 'Minor salivary gland biopsy in neonatal hemochromatosis', Archives of otolaryngology--head & neck surgery, 130(6), 760-3.

Soll, R. F. (2010) 'Probiotics: are we ready for routine use?', Pediatrics, 125(5), 1071-2.

Spencer, A. U., Neaga, A., West, B., Safran, J., Brown, P., Btaiche, I., Kuzma-O'Reilly, B. and Teitelbaum, D. H. (2005) 'Pediatric short bowel syndrome: redefining predictors of success', Ann Surg, 242(3), 403-9; discussion 409-12.

Stoll, B. J., Hansen, N. I., Bell, E. F., Shankaran, S., Laptook, A. R., Walsh, M. C., Hale, E. C., Newman, N. S., Schibler, K., Carlo, W. A., Kennedy, K. A., Poindexter, B. B., Finer, N. N., Ehrenkranz, R. A.,

Sundaram, S. S., Alonso, E. M. and Whitington, P. F. (2003) 'Liver transplantation in neonates', Liver transplantation : official publication of the American Association for the Study of Liver Diseases and the International Liver Transplantation Society, 9(8), 783-8.

Tarnow-Mordi, W. O., Wilkinson, D., Trivedi, A. and Brok, J. (2010) 'Probiotics reduce all-cause mortality and necrotizing enterocolitis: it is time to change practice', Pediatrics, 125(5), 1068-70.

te Braake, F. W., van den Akker, C. H., Riedijk, M. A. and van Goudoever, J. B. (2007) 'Parenteral amino acid and energy administration to premature infants in early life', Seminars in fetal & neonatal medicine, 12(1), 11-8.

Thorn, S. R., Rozance, P. J., Brown, L. D., & Hay, W. W., Jr. (2011). The intrauterine growth restriction phenotype: fetal adaptations and potential implications for later life insulin resistance and diabetes. *Semin Reprod Med, 29*(3), 225-236. doi: 10.1055/s-0031-1275516.

Timpani, G., Foti, F., Nicolo, A., Nicotina, P. A., Nicastro, E. and Iorio, R. (2007) 'Is exchange transfusion a possible treatment for neonatal hemochromatosis?', Journal of hepatology, 47(5), 732-5.

Touloukian, R. J. and Smith, G. J. (1983) 'Normal intestinal length in preterm infants', J Pediatr Surg, 18(6), 720-3.

Tsai, A., Paltiel, H. J., Sena, L. M., Kim, H. B., Fishman, S. J. and Alomari, A. I. (2009) 'Neonatal hemochromatosis and patent ductus venosus: clinical course and diagnostic pitfalls', Pediatric radiology, 39(8), 823-7.

Tsang R, Uauy R, Koletzko B and Zlotkin, S. (2005) Consensus recommendations; summary of reasonable nutrient intakes for preterm infants. , In: Nutrition of the Preterm Infant. Scientific Basis and Practical Guidelines. Digital Publishing Inc; Cincinnati, Ohio.

Vohr, B. R., Poindexter, B. B., Dusick, A. M., McKinley, L. T., Wright, L. L., Langer, J. C. and Poole, W. K. (2006) 'Beneficial effects of breast milk in the neonatal intensive care unit on the developmental outcome of extremely low birth weight infants at 18 months of age', Pediatrics, 118(1), e115-23.

von Berg, A., Filipiak-Pittroff, B., Kramer, U., Link, E., Bollrath, C., Brockow, I., Koletzko, S., Grubl, A., Heinrich, J., Wichmann, H. E., Bauer, C. P., Reinhardt, D. and Berdel, D. (2008) 'Preventive effect of hydrolyzed infant formulas persists until age 6 years: long-term results from the German Infant Nutritional Intervention Study (GINI)', The Journal of allergy and clinical immunology, 121(6), 1442-7.

Vossbeck, S., de Camargo, O. K., Grab, D., Bode, H., & Pohlandt, F. (2001). Neonatal and neurodevelopmental outcome in infants born before 30 weeks of gestation with absent or reversed end-diastolic flow velocities in the umbilical artery. *Eur J Pediatr, 160*(2), 128-134.

Wadhawan, R., Oh, W., Perritt, R., Laptook, A. R., Poole, K., Wright, L. L., Fanaroff, A. A., Duara, S., Stoll, B. J. and Goldberg, R. (2007) 'Association between early postnatal weight loss and death or BPD in small and appropriate for gestational age extremely low-birth-weight infants', J Perinatol, 27(6), 359-64.

Wales, P. W. and Christison-Lagay, E. R. (2010) 'Short bowel syndrome: epidemiology and etiology', Semin Pediatr Surg, 19(1), 3-9.

Wales, P. W., de Silva, N., Kim, J. H., Lecce, L., Sandhu, A. and Moore, A. M. (2005) 'Neonatal short bowel syndrome: a cohort study', J Pediatr Surg, 40(5), 755-62.

Wales, P. W., Kosar, C., Carricato, M., de Silva, N., Lang, K. and Avitzur, Y. (2011) 'Ethanol lock therapy to reduce the incidence of catheter-related bloodstream infections in home parenteral nutrition patients with intestinal failure: preliminary experience', J Pediatr Surg, 46(5), 951-6.

Whitington, P. F. (2007) 'Neonatal hemochromatosis: a congenital alloimmune hepatitis', Seminars in liver disease, 27(3), 243-50.

Whitington, P. F. and Kelly, S. (2008) 'Outcome of pregnancies at risk for neonatal hemochromatosis is improved by treatment with high-dose intravenous immunoglobulin', Pediatrics, 121(6), e1615-21.

WHO (2006) 'WHO Multicentre Growth Reference Study', Acta Paediatr Suppl, 450, 5-101.

Wienerroither, H., Steiner, H., Tomaselli, J., Lobendanz, M., & Thun-Hohenstein, L. (2001). Intrauterine blood flow and long-term intellectual, neurologic, and social development. *Obstet Gynecol, 97*(3), 449-453.

Williams, H. (2007) 'Green for danger! Intestinal malrotation and volvulus', *Arch Dis Child Educ Pract Ed*, 92(3), ep87-91.

Williams, H., McKiernan, P., Kelly, D. and Baumann, U. (2006) 'Magnetic resonance imaging in neonatal hemochromatosis--are we there yet?', Liver transplantation : official publication of the American Association for the Study of Liver Diseases and the International Liver Transplantation Society, 12(11), 1725.

Williams, R. L., Creasy, R. K., Cunningham, G. C., Hawes, W. E., Norris, F. D., & Tashiro, M. (1982). Fetal growth and perinatal viability in California. *Obstet Gynecol, 59*(5), 624-632.

Wilson, D. C., Cairns, P., Halliday, H. L., Reid, M., McClure, G. and Dodge, J. A. (1997) 'Randomised controlled trial of an aggressive nutritional regimen in sick very low birthweight infants', Archives of disease in childhood. Fetal and neonatal edition, 77(1), F4-11.

Yeung, M. Y. (2006) 'Postnatal growth, neurodevelopment and altered adiposity after preterm birth--from a clinical nutrition perspective', Acta paediatrica, 95(8), 909-17.

Zarrough, A. E., Srinivasan, S. K. & Wulkan, M. L. (2010) 'Incidental chylous fluid during hernia repair may be a harbinger of malrotation', *J Pediatr Surg, 45(1)* E17-8.

4

Brain Injury in Preterm Infants

Zoe Iliodromiti[1], Dimitrios Zygouris[2], Paraskevi Karagianni[3], Panagiotis Belitsos[4], Angelos Daniilidis[5] and Nikolaos Vrachnis[6]

[1]Neonatal Unit, 2nd Department of Obstetrics and Gynecology, University of Athens Medical School, Aretaieio Hospital, Athens,

[2]3nd Department of Obstetrics and Gynecology, University of Athens Medical School, Attiko Hospital, Athens,

[3]2nd NICU and Neonatology Department, Aristotle University of Thessaloniki, General Papageorgiou Hospital, Thessaloniki,

[4]Department of Obstetrics and Gynecology, Chalkida Hospital, Evia,

[5]Department of Obstetrics and Gynecology, University of Thessaloniki Medical School, Ippokrateio Hospital, Thessaloniki,

[6]2nd Department of Obstetrics and Gynecology, University of Athens Medical School, Aretaieio Hospital, Athens,

Greece

1. Introduction

It is well known that the number of surviving preterm infants is today steadily on the increase (Fanaroff, Stoll et al. 2007). Nevertheless, despite the improvements in perinatal medicine, brain injury is still a major clinical problem and remains a significant cause of perinatal morbidity and mortality (Volpe 2009). Moreover, the numerous environmental factors to which the fetal brain is exposed during fetal development, additionally linked to factors of a genetic origin, not only subject the infant to the severe risk of morbidity and mortality, but can also lead to a wide spectrum of functional and behavioral disorders throughout the individual's life.

Recent studies have demonstrated that cognitive and behavioral deficits are significantly higher in preterm neonates (Burd, Chai et al. 2009; Burd, Bentz et al. 2010). Also reported, as concerns long-term consequences, are higher rates of educational difficulties, epileptic seizures, visual damages and reduction in the mean intelligence quotient (Hack 2006). The biggest problem in preterm infants is damage to white matter. This damage involves multifocal necrosis resulting in cystic periventricular leukomalacia (PVL) or a diffuse astrogliosis and loss of myelin-producing oligodendrocytes. Maternal infection and inflammation during pregnancy may also lead to development of cerebral palsy (CP) and, less commonly, to other neuropsychiatric disorders (Yoon, Romero et al. 2000; Wu 2002; Meyer, Feldon et al. 2006; Meyer, Nyffeler et al. 2006). The final result is not only the great distress incurred by the newborn and later the child and adult, but also the considerable burden inflicted on both their families and the national health system.

Although there are a large number of clinical and experimental studies which seek to describe the exact pathophysiologic mechanism involved in perinatal brain injury, this is not as yet completely understood. Further investigation is highly likely to yield pharmaceutical intervention that will achieve prevention or resolution of preterm brain injury.

2. Pathological aspects of preterm brain injury

The most prominent pathological characteristic in brain injury is white matter damage, especially in the periventicular tracts such as PVL (Periventicular Leukomalacia). The damage consists of necrotic areas, with the severe type, namely cystic PVL, being characterized by astrogliosis and microgliosis. However, the incidence of cystic PVL is today ever more rarely encountered due to contemporary advanced perinatal care: nowadays it concerns less than 5% of all cases, (Inder, Warfield et al. 2005) the majority of these involving diffuse cellular loss without any cystic establishment. This damage is referred to as non-cystic PVL and is characterized solely by diffuse necrosis accompanied by activated microglia and reactive astrocytes. Furthermore, in about one third of PVL cases neuronal loss and gliosis in the basal ganglia and dentate cerebellar nuclei (Pierson, Folkerth et al. 2007) and thalamus were detected (Ligam, Haynes et al. 2009).

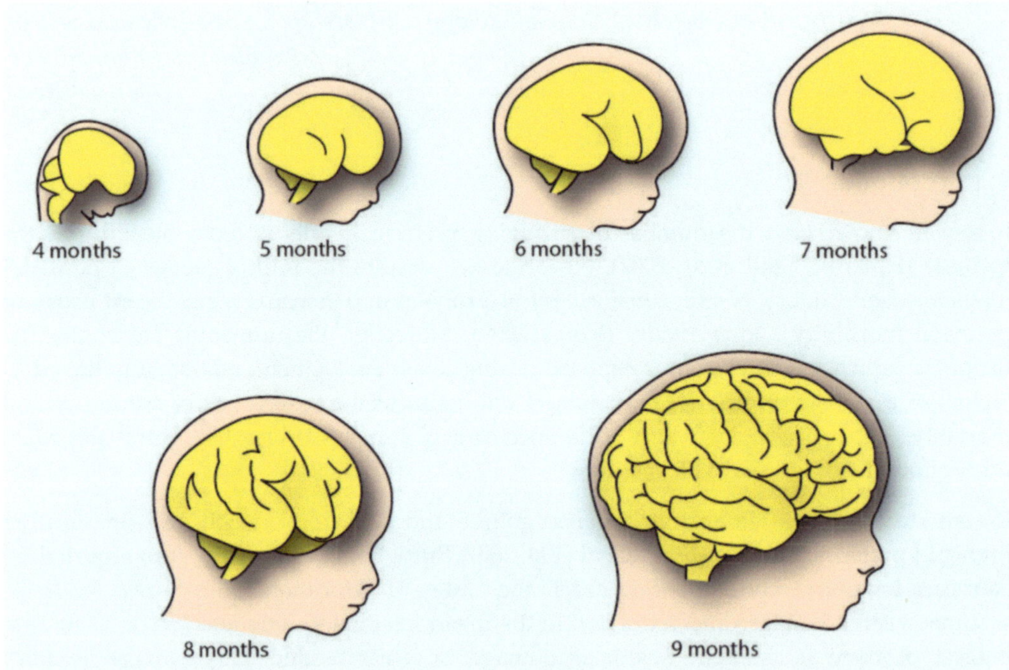

Fig. 1. Development of fetal brain. The third through the ninth month is the fetal stage, while the fourth month marks the beginning of the fetus' motor function. The commissures of brain develop at this stage and the ventricular system is completed. Cerebellar development begins by the sixth month and is completed two years after birth. However, the first eight weeks, defined as the embryonic period, are also crucial for normal brain development. The cerebral hemispheres differentiate around the fifth week, by the end of which period the cerebral cortex has undergone great growth and development.

PVL frequently exists together with intraventricular hemorrhages, this reflecting the vulnerability of the premyelinating oligodendrocytes (Pre-Ols) (Back, Luo et al. 2005). Injury to white matter is most thoroughly investigated via ultrasound and magnetic resonance imaging (MRI), the latter method clearly demonstrating a volume reduction of the thalamus and basal ganglia (Inder, Anderson et al. 2003; Inder, Warfield et al. 2005), the hippocampus (Isaacs, Lucas et al. 2000) and the cerebellum (Allin, Matsumoto et al. 2001).

The fact that injury of grey matter is also a crucial component of preterm brain injury is an additional finding derived from MRI studies (Peterson, Vohr et al. 2000; Lin, Okumura et al. 2001; Woodward, Anderson et al. 2006), which revealed a long-term reduction of gray matter volume and an association between white matter injury and reduction of gray matter volume (Woodward, Anderson et al. 2006). Interestingly, recent data show that the same injury may also be established in term infants (Iwata, Bainbridge et al. 2010).

Brain development in the perinatal period is adjusted by a crucial balance of apoptosis and survival of cerebral cells. In about 70% of the cases the brain injury is established in the early hours and predicts the long-term outcome (Hayakawa, Okumura et al. 1999; Kubota, Okumura et al. 2002). It seems that there an increase in cell death that causes a crucial loss of the developing brain cell population. The result of this acute neuronal damage will be partly reflected in chronic anatomical deficits, as clinical brain injury develops gradually.

2.1 Glial cells: A protective network in the fetal brain

Glial cells form a defensive network that shields the brain parenchyma, participating in protection, repair and regeneration of damaged neurons during injury or disease (Peterson, Vohr et al. 2000). This network consists of microglia and astrocytes and also plays an important role in removal of dead neurons and inflammatory products.

Microglia, the primary component, penetrates the brain tissue during fetal development and removes the dead neural cells and the toxic deposits that have accumulated, this being a cornerstone function of these vital resident macrophages during neurodevelopment.

Astrocytes are the second major type of glial cells, which have varied influence on epithelial cells. They increase the blood-brain barrier (Girvin, Gordon et al. 2002) and, by activating the circulating T-cells, they regulate the immune response and homeostasis of the fetal brain. This regulation is achieved by secretion of pro- and anti-inflammatory cytokines such as interleukins (IL) and tumor necrosis factor-α (TNF-α).

The main causes of perinatal brain injury are ischemic injury, glutamate injury, cytokine-associated intrauterine infection and inflammation, and cerebral hemorrhage.

3.1 The role of hypoxia / ischemia in brain injury

Nowadays, perinatal hypoxia occurs at a low rate in preterm infants. It nonetheless remains a major problem that is substantially higher in preterm (73 / 1000 live births) than in full term infants (25 / 1000 live births) (Low 2004). Preterm infants are found to be less susceptible than term infants to developing brain injury after fetal hypoxemia (Gunn, Quaedackers et al. 2001). Although the autoregulatory mechanisms of cerebral blood flow are established very early in pregnancy and work efficiently, even in very immature infants with reduced blood supply, adequate oxygen and glucose supply, essential for the normal functioning and development of the fetal brain, drop either acutely or gradually during intrauterine life, occlusion of the umbilical cord being the main acute cause, with placental insufficiency resulting in chronic blood hypoperfusion. Whatever is the cause of fetal hypoxemia, it results in severe brain injury (Volpe 2009). However, the exact degree of hypoxia that leads to irreversible brain damage has not as yet been determined. The fetal brain has the ability to react in hypoxia by increasing the cerebral blood flow via reflex vasodilatation (Pearce 2006). Moreover, always to be borne in mind is the anatomical vulnerability and relative vulnerability of different areas and populations of oligodendronglia in white matter. This factor would appear to explain recent experimental data that were unable to account for cerebral ischemia by differences in local blood flow.

While postnatal blood pressure has also been regarded as a marker of the induced brain injury, in many studies no relationship was found between hypotension in preterm infants and neurological defects (CPL, CP) (Trounce, Shaw et al. 1988; Perlman, Risser et al. 1996; Cunningham, Symon et al. 1999; Dammann, Allred et al. 2002). Systemic hypotension alone was associated with neurological defects by other researchers (Low, Froese et al. 1993; Murphy, Hope et al. 1997; Martens, Rijken et al. 2003), a discrepancy that can easily be explained by the fact that blood pressure is not a reliable marker of the possible impaired cardiac output and the subsequent cerebral perfusion.

The fact that the crucial moment at which hypoxemia causes brain injury has not yet been defined presents a major diagnostic problem. Moreover, it is still controversial whether brain injury can be induced by hypoxemia alone or whether it arises from a combination of other simultaneous pathophysiological factors.

3.2 Glutamate-induced brain injury

Glutamate is the major excitatory transmitter in the brain and is involved in the majority of the aspects of normal brain function, such as memory, cognition and learning. It is connected to postsynaptic glutamate receptors, its connection to and subsequent activation of these receptors leading to an increase of the free intracellular calcium. This last activates high levels of proteases, endonucleases and lipase enzymes, thus ultimately bringing about cellular death. In addition to activation of proteases, protein synthesis is inhibited as a result of brain hypoxia.

Experimental data show a wide variability in the distribution and composition of the glutamate receptors in the Central Nervous System (CNS), (McDonald, Johnston et al. 1990), this explaining why there is no clear correlation between brain cellular death and glutamate levels (Mitani, Andou et al. 1992). Nevertheless, glutamate, the cornerstone of hypoxia-induced brain injury, plays a highly toxic role, especially with regard to white matter in preterm neonates. Glutamate is produced by the developing oligodendrocytes and axons (Rossi, Oshima et al. 2000; Desilva, Kinney et al. 2007) and is highly toxic in vitro (Choi 1992). Moreover, it renders even more vulnerable the premyelinating oligodendrocytes, though not the mature cells (Itoh, Beesley et al. 2002).

Despite the above in vitro data, it has not thus far been definitively established in vivo that hypoxia results in high and thus toxic concentrations of glutamate. Furthermore, a recent study did not demonstrate any increase in the extracellular glutamate levels in white matter after cerebral hypoxia (Fraser, Bennet et al. 2008). It seems that the extracellular levels of calcium rise significantly in gray matter (Henderson, Reynolds et al. 1998; Loeliger, Watson et al. 2003; Dohmen, Kumura et al. 2005) in contrast to white matter, where the rise is minimal and declines rapidly.

3.3 Reactive Oxygen Species (ROS) and Reactive Nitrogen Species (RNS)

Oxygen radicals are produced in large amounts after excessive tissue ischemia. In cerebral tissue this is carried out via activation of superoxide dismutase, xanthine oxidase and caspace-9. This activation leads to DNA fragmentation, destruction of the cellular membranes and various degrees of cell damage, eventually resulting in cell death (Davies and Goldberg 1987). Moreover, ischemia in brain tissue induces metabolism of arachidonic acid, causing further production of ROS.

A large number of experimental studies have demonstrated the severe impact of oxygen radicals on brain injury. Immature oligodendroglia, in contrast to mature cells, seems much more vulnerable to ROS (Back, Gan et al. 1998). Furthermore, the use of allopurinol (an inhibitor of xanthine oxidase) seems to have a protective effect on cerebral tissue, some studies demonstrating that the neuronal loss was completely inhibited (Palmer, Towfighi et al. 1993). Another study showed that after induced cerebral hypoxia the cerebral ascorbyl radical was increased, leading to white matter injury (Welin, Sandberg et al. 2005). In contrast, in preterm fetal sheep there was no increase of ROS in the periventricular white matter (Desilva, Kinney et al. 2007). It thus appears evident that the receptor-mediated toxicity alone plays a major role in PVL, as excitatory acid levels do not increase even in cases of severe ischemia (Rosin, Bates et al. 2004).

Nitric oxide, also known as nitrogen monoxide (NO), is another free radical implicated in tissue ischemia. During cerebral ischemia, an excessive increase of intracellular calcium takes place, activating the NO-synthetase. The latter enzyme produces NO, which also induces the toxicity of the other oxygen radicals, such as superoxide radicals and hydroxyl radicals. Inhibition of NO-synthetase in animal models was shown to be highly protective in ischemic neural tissue (Hamada, Hayakawa et al. 1994), reducing hippocampal and cortical damage (Ferriero, Holtzman et al. 1996).

3.4 Intrauterine infection / inflammation

Intrauterine infection/inflammation is a major cause of fetal organ dysfunctions in the perinatal period and the fetal brain is one of the most vulnerable organs. Inflammation is a major factor in preterm and term delivered infants (Malamitsi-Puchner, Vrachnis et al. 2006) with regard to perinatal brain damage, including CP (Dammann and Leviton 1997; Volpe 2009). Intrauterine inflammation may lead to fetal inflammatory response syndrome (FIRS), clinical chorioamnionitis or clinically silent histological chorioamnionitis (Vrachnis, Vitoratos et al. 2010). Recent clinical data suggest that inflammatory response in brain tissue is the most significant mechanism causing brain injury. Inflammation reduces brain weight and volume as a result of destruction of white matter, the main loss being found at the level of the lateral ventricles and around the foramen of Monro. Modern neuro-imaging techniques have enabled identification of the foci of necrosis in the white matter around the lateral ventricle, while an inhibition of myelination and astrocytosis after intrauterine infection has also been observed.

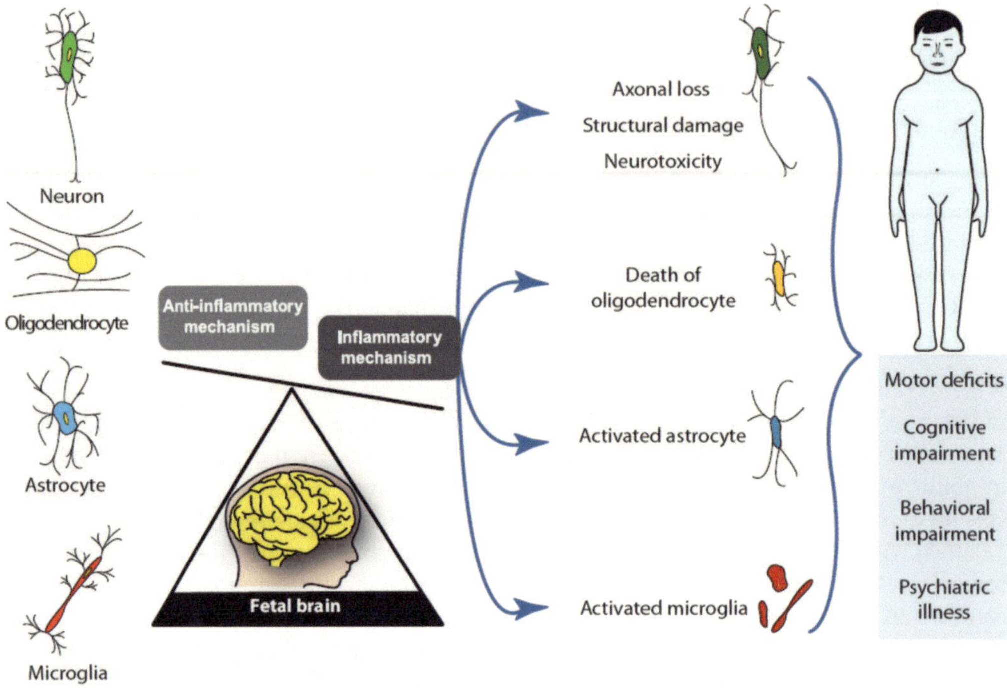

Fig. 2. Mechanisms of brain injury in preterm neonates. Chorioamnionitis is the prime factor triggering the inflammation cascade in the fetal brain, contributing to the pathogenesis of brain injury. Activated asrocytes and microglia play a cornerstone role in white matter damage, leading to functional and behavioral disorders throughout the individual's life.

Proinflammatory cytokines have been found significantly elevated in the amniotic fluid and fetal brain of neonates with infection, including local inflammatory response leading to brain injury (Yoon, Romero et al. 2000; Kadhim, Tabarki et al. 2001). Elevated levels of cytokines have additionally been observed in the amniotic fluid and blood of neonates that developed cerebral palsy (Yoon, Jun et al. 1997; Nelson, Dambrosia et al. 1998). FIRS has also been associated with increased levels of IL-6, IL-8 and TNF-α and implicated in white matter injury and predominantly in PVL development, resulting in later motor and cognitive impairments. In cases of confirmed PVL it was found that the high levels of IL-1b and TNF-α were detected even from the early stage of the injury, up until the late stage of cystic PVL (Kadhim, Tabarki et al. 2001). Moreover, autopsy studies of PVL cases revealed very high levels of TNF-α and hypertrophic astrocytes in the areas of damaged white matter (Deguchi, Oguchi et al. 1997). Experimental data show that lipopolysacharide (LPS) infection induces TNF-α production from astrocytes and may also cause severe decentralization of fetal circulation, resulting in cerebral hypoperfusion and subsequent ischemic brain injury. Another study showed that in almost 90% of the PVL cases TNF-α, IL-1 and IL-6 were highly expressed (Yoon, Jun et al. 1997). These data are in agreement with the finding that IL-1β induces in vitro microglial activation (Hailer, Vogt et al. 2005). Activated microglia additionally produce TNF-α IL-1b, inducing apoptosis of oligodentrocytes and their progenitors.

Other inflammatory cytokines, such as IL-12, IL-15 and IL-18, were also found in children with CP (Zupan, Gonzalez et al. 1996). IL-18 is activated by caspase-1 and causes the subsequent production of IL-1, TNF-α and interferon-γ. As a result, IL-18 induces apoptosis and is associated with development of neonatal PVL and CP (Keelan, Blumenstein et al. 2003). IL-18 was found in higher concentrations in vulnerable animal models, indicating its potentially important role in the establishment of brain injury (Hedtjarn, Leverin et al. 2002; Hedtjarn, Mallard et al. 2005).

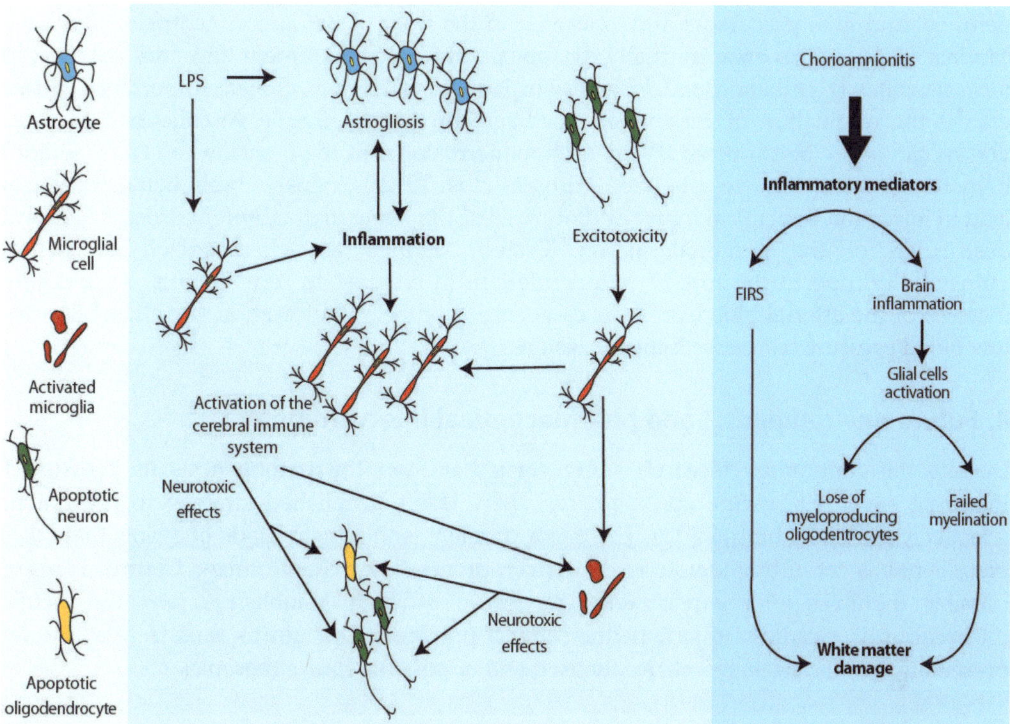

Fig. 3. Molecular pathways leading from intrauterine inflammation to brain injury. Intrauterine infection by LPS induces astrogliosis and inflammation through microglial cells, which subsequently triggers oligodendrocyte apoptosis through inflammatory cytokines such as IL-1β, IL-6, IL-8, and TNF-α and reactive oxygen species. NF-κβ activation by intrauterine inflammation additionally results in overexpression of TNF-α, IL-1β, IL-6 and IL-8. This inflammatory cascade results in fetal inflammatory response syndrome (FIRS) or local brain inflammation and finally damage of white matter.

Furthermore, activation of Toll-Like Receptors (TLRs) was found to participate in the intrauterine infection/inflammation that induces inflammatory response and damage in brain tissue (Yuan, Sun et al. 2010). TLRs, membrane-bound proteins used by cells of the innate immune system, play a vital role in the immune response of the central nervous system, their activation in the immune process concerning TLR_1, TLR_2, TLR_3, and especially TLR_6 receptors (Abrahams, Aldo et al. 2008). The activated TLRs receptors induce Nuclear

Factor-kappa β (NF-κβ) production, leading to induction of NO expression in the brain (Chen, Ho et al. 2005). NF-κβ is also activated by proinflammatory cytokines after exposure to LPS and thereafter induces the expression of TNF-α, IL-1β, IL-6 and IL-8 (Belt, Baldassare et al. 1999).

3.5 Cerebral hemorrhage causing brain injury

In preterm infants cerebral hemorrhage, mainly peri- and intra-ventricular, is a common finding. In the developing fetal brain the germinal matrix is the main area of proliferation of neuronal and glial precursors and is located in the floor of the lateral ventricle, above the caudate nucleus. This area gradually disappears during development and does not exist in term neonates (Hambleton and Wigglesworth 1976). The great clinical importance of this area is the origination of cerebral hemorrhage through its fragile vascular net, as these vessels can easily be ruptured. Perinatal hypoperfusion and hypotension can cause a rapid hemorrhage from these vessels (Tan, Williams et al. 1992). Extensive brain hemorrhage can lead to infraction ischemical injury and necrosis of the white matter, and hydrocephalus and destruction of the germinal matrix. Preterm fetuses are characterized by neural vulnerability, due to the loss of autoregulation, in contrast to term infants. As a result, increase of the arterial blood pressure can cause rupture in the cerebral vessels, while very low blood pressure can cause ischemic lesions.

4. Future environmental and pharmaceutical interventions

Despite the continuous research being carried out on the pathogenesis of a disorder incurring such very severe consequences, there is no established strategy to prevent or effectively treat fetal brain injury. The major problem is that the cascade of events that takes place is not as yet fully understood. Moreover, proceeding to Randomized Control Trials of possible therapies after experimental results in order to establish a new therapeutic intervention is, needless to say, neither ethical nor legal. Our aim is thus to offer a brief presentation of the strategies currently used and of possible future therapies.

4.1 Hypothermia

A recent meta-analysis (Edwards, Brocklehurst et al. 2010) confirmed the neuroprotective effect of moderate hypothermia, while experimental studies on adult animals show that lowering the brain temperature results in reducing neuronal cell damage (Berger, Jensen et al. 1998; Gunn, Gunn et al. 1998; Garnier, Pfeiffer et al. 2001). However, this procedure does not seem to be fully protective in the injured brain, as it does not induce the neuronal repair that is essential for normal neurodevelopment. The clinical data have merely demonstrated that mild hypothermia is not harmful in infants with perinatal asphyxia, but there was no obvious benefit (Gunn, Gluckman et al. 1998; Azzopardi, Robertson et al. 2000).

4.2 Other potential pharmacological interventions

We have already described above the crucial role of glutamate and reactive oxygen and nitrogen species in the pathogenesis of brain injury. Today, glutamate antagonists and NO inhibitors are being experimentally used to prevent cellular death. Flunarizine is an antagonist of calcium channels and has been utilized (Garnier, Berger et al. 1998) in sheep models for protection of the fetal brain from ischemic injury, while erythropoietin is also under investigation for its anti-inflammatory, anti-oxidant and neurotrophic action (Campana and Myers 2001) in brain ischemia. Melatonin is another possible therapy as it additionally has an anti-oxidant effect and crosses the placental and blood-brain barrier (Reiter, Tan et al. 2000). It has been proposed (Gitto, Pellegrino et al. 2009) for clinical use during the perinatal period for reduction of oxidative stress (Fulia, Gitto et al. 2001). Finally, a retrospective analysis (Nelson and Grether 1995) showed that application of magnesium significantly decreased the incidence of cerebral palsy.

5. Conclusion

In conclusion, despite the numerous experimental and clinical studies that are ongoing, there is still much debate as to the exact mechanism of brain injury in preterm infants. Further research is needed to clarify the precise part played by intrauterine inflammation and oxygen and nitrogen radicals. Because the role of glutamate is undeniable in brain injury, glutamate inhibition appears to have a promising future in brain injury intervention. Furthermore, the development of therapies targeting astrocytes and activated microglia opens up yet another potential approach. Thus, while to date hypothermia is the sole established therapy, it is clear that future research will focus on a combination of therapies taking into account both pharmacological and molecular factors for the creation of an improved extrauterine environment for preterm infants.

6. References

Abrahams, V. M., P. B. Aldo, et al. (2008). "TLR6 modulates first trimester trophoblast responses to peptidoglycan." J Immunol 180(9): 6035-6043.

Allin, M., H. Matsumoto, et al. (2001). "Cognitive and motor function and the size of the cerebellum in adolescents born very pre-term." Brain 124(Pt 1): 60-66.

Azzopardi, D., N. J. Robertson, et al. (2000). "Pilot study of treatment with whole body hypothermia for neonatal encephalopathy." Pediatrics 106(4): 684-694.

Back, S. A., X. Gan, et al. (1998). "Maturation-dependent vulnerability of oligodendrocytes to oxidative stress-induced death caused by glutathione depletion." J Neurosci 18(16): 6241-6253.

Back, S. A., N. L. Luo, et al. (2005). "Selective vulnerability of preterm white matter to oxidative damage defined by F2-isoprostanes." Ann Neurol 58(1): 108-120.

Belt, A. R., J. J. Baldassare, et al. (1999). "The nuclear transcription factor NF-kappaB mediates interleukin-1beta-induced expression of cyclooxygenase-2 in human myometrial cells." Am J Obstet Gynecol 181(2): 359-366.

Berger, R., A. Jensen, et al. (1998). "Effect of mild hypothermia during and after transient in vitro ischemia on metabolic disturbances in hippocampal slices at different stages of development." Brain Res Dev Brain Res 105(1): 67-77.

Burd, I., A. I. Bentz, et al. (2010). "Inflammation-induced preterm birth alters neuronal morphology in the mouse fetal brain." J Neurosci Res 88(9): 1872-1881.

Burd, I., J. Chai, et al. (2009). "Beyond white matter damage: fetal neuronal injury in a mouse model of preterm birth." Am J Obstet Gynecol 201(3): 279 e271-278.

Campana, W. M. and R. R. Myers (2001). "Erythropoietin and erythropoietin receptors in the peripheral nervous system: changes after nerve injury." FASEB J 15(10): 1804-1806.

Chen, J. C., F. M. Ho, et al. (2005). "Inhibition of iNOS gene expression by quercetin is mediated by the inhibition of IkappaB kinase, nuclear factor-kappa B and STAT1, and depends on heme oxygenase-1 induction in mouse BV-2 microglia." Eur J Pharmacol 521(1-3): 9-20.

Choi, D. W. (1992). "Excitotoxic cell death." J Neurobiol 23(9): 1261-1276.

Cunningham, S., A. G. Symon, et al. (1999). "Intra-arterial blood pressure reference ranges, death and morbidity in very low birthweight infants during the first seven days of life." Early Hum Dev 56(2-3): 151-165.

Dammann, O., E. N. Allred, et al. (2002). "Systemic hypotension and white-matter damage in preterm infants." Dev Med Child Neurol 44(2): 82-90.

Dammann, O. and A. Leviton (1997). "Maternal intrauterine infection, cytokines, and brain damage in the preterm newborn." Pediatr Res 42(1): 1-8.

Davies, K. J. and A. L. Goldberg (1987). "Oxygen radicals stimulate intracellular proteolysis and lipid peroxidation by independent mechanisms in erythrocytes." J Biol Chem 262(17): 8220-8226.

Deguchi, K., K. Oguchi, et al. (1997). "Characteristic neuropathology of leukomalacia in extremely low birth weight infants." Pediatr Neurol 16(4): 296-300.

Desilva, T. M., H. C. Kinney, et al. (2007). "The glutamate transporter EAAT2 is transiently expressed in developing human cerebral white matter." J Comp Neurol 501(6): 879-890.

Dohmen, C., E. Kumura, et al. (2005). "Extracellular correlates of glutamate toxicity in short-term cerebral ischemia and reperfusion: a direct in vivo comparison between white and gray matter." Brain Res 1037(1-2): 43-51.

Edwards, A. D., P. Brocklehurst, et al. (2010). "Neurological outcomes at 18 months of age after moderate hypothermia for perinatal hypoxic ischaemic encephalopathy: synthesis and meta-analysis of trial data." BMJ 340: c363.

Fanaroff, A. A., B. J. Stoll, et al. (2007). "Trends in neonatal morbidity and mortality for very low birthweight infants." Am J Obstet Gynecol 196(2): 147 e141-148.

Ferriero, D. M., D. M. Holtzman, et al. (1996). "Neonatal mice lacking neuronal nitric oxide synthase are less vulnerable to hypoxic-ischemic injury." Neurobiol Dis 3(1): 64-71.

Fraser, M., L. Bennet, et al. (2008). "Extracellular amino acids and lipid peroxidation products in periventricular white matter during and after cerebral ischemia in preterm fetal sheep." J Neurochem 105(6): 2214-2223.

Fulia, F., E. Gitto, et al. (2001). "Increased levels of malondialdehyde and nitrite/nitrate in the blood of asphyxiated newborns: reduction by melatonin." J Pineal Res 31(4): 343-349.

Garnier, Y., R. Berger, et al. (1998). "Low-dose flunarizine does not affect short-term fetal circulatory responses to acute asphyxia in sheep near term." Reprod Fertil Dev 10(5): 405-411.

Garnier, Y., D. Pfeiffer, et al. (2001). "Effects of mild hypothermia on metabolic disturbances in fetal hippocampal slices after oxygen/glucose deprivation depend on depth and time delay of cooling." J Soc Gynecol Investig 8(4): 198-205.

Girvin, A. M., K. B. Gordon, et al. (2002). "Differential abilities of central nervous system resident endothelial cells and astrocytes to serve as inducible antigen-presenting cells." Blood 99(10): 3692-3701.

Gitto, E., S. Pellegrino, et al. (2009). "Oxidative stress of the newborn in the pre- and postnatal period and the clinical utility of melatonin." J Pineal Res 46(2): 128-139.

Gunn, A. J., P. D. Gluckman, et al. (1998). "Selective head cooling in newborn infants after perinatal asphyxia: a safety study." Pediatrics 102(4 Pt 1): 885-892.

Gunn, A. J., T. R. Gunn, et al. (1998). "Neuroprotection with prolonged head cooling started before postischemic seizures in fetal sheep." Pediatrics 102(5): 1098-1106.

Gunn, A. J., J. S. Quaedackers, et al. (2001). "The premature fetus: not as defenseless as we thought, but still paradoxically vulnerable?" Dev Neurosci 23(3): 175-179.

Hack, M. (2006). "Young adult outcomes of very-low-birth-weight children." Semin Fetal Neonatal Med 11(2): 127-137.

Hailer, N. P., C. Vogt, et al. (2005). "Interleukin-1beta exacerbates and interleukin-1 receptor antagonist attenuates neuronal injury and microglial activation after excitotoxic damage in organotypic hippocampal slice cultures." Eur J Neurosci 21(9): 2347-2360.

Hamada, Y., T. Hayakawa, et al. (1994). "Inhibitor of nitric oxide synthesis reduces hypoxic-ischemic brain damage in the neonatal rat." Pediatr Res 35(1): 10-14.

Hambleton, G. and J. S. Wigglesworth (1976). "Origin of intraventricular haemorrhage in the preterm infant." Arch Dis Child 51(9): 651-659.

Hayakawa, F., A. Okumura, et al. (1999). "Determination of timing of brain injury in preterm infants with periventricular leukomalacia with serial neonatal electroencephalography." Pediatrics 104(5 Pt 1): 1077-1081.

Hedtjarn, M., A. L. Leverin, et al. (2002). "Interleukin-18 involvement in hypoxic-ischemic brain injury." J Neurosci 22(14): 5910-5919.

Hedtjarn, M., C. Mallard, et al. (2005). "White matter injury in the immature brain: role of interleukin-18." Neurosci Lett 373(1): 16-20.

Henderson, J. L., J. D. Reynolds, et al. (1998). "Chronic hypoxemia causes extracellular glutamate concentration to increase in the cerebral cortex of the near-term fetal sheep." Brain Res Dev Brain Res 105(2): 287-293.

Inder, T. E., N. J. Anderson, et al. (2003). "White matter injury in the premature infant: a comparison between serial cranial sonographic and MR findings at term." AJNR Am J Neuroradiol 24(5): 805-809.

Inder, T. E., S. K. Warfield, et al. (2005). "Abnormal cerebral structure is present at term in premature infants." Pediatrics 115(2): 286-294.

Isaacs, E. B., A. Lucas, et al. (2000). "Hippocampal volume and everyday memory in children of very low birth weight." Pediatr Res 47(6): 713-720.

Itoh, T., J. Beesley, et al. (2002). "AMPA glutamate receptor-mediated calcium signaling is transiently enhanced during development of oligodendrocytes." J Neurochem 81(2): 390-402.

Iwata, S., A. Bainbridge, et al. (2010). "Subtle white matter injury is common in term-born infants with a wide range of risks." Int J Dev Neurosci 28(7): 573-580.

Kadhim, H., B. Tabarki, et al. (2001). "Inflammatory cytokines in the pathogenesis of periventricular leukomalacia." Neurology 56(10): 1278-1284.

Keelan, J. A., M. Blumenstein, et al. (2003). "Cytokines, prostaglandins and parturition--a review." Placenta 24 Suppl A: S33-46.

Kubota, T., A. Okumura, et al. (2002). "Combination of neonatal electroencephalography and ultrasonography: sensitive means of early diagnosis of periventricular leukomalacia." Brain Dev 24(7): 698-702.

Ligam, P., R. L. Haynes, et al. (2009). "Thalamic damage in periventricular leukomalacia: novel pathologic observations relevant to cognitive deficits in survivors of prematurity." Pediatr Res 65(5): 524-529.

Lin, Y., A. Okumura, et al. (2001). "Quantitative evaluation of thalami and basal ganglia in infants with periventricular leukomalacia." Dev Med Child Neurol 43(7): 481-485.

Loeliger, M., C. S. Watson, et al. (2003). "Extracellular glutamate levels and neuropathology in cerebral white matter following repeated umbilical cord occlusion in the near term fetal sheep." Neuroscience 116(3): 705-714.

Low, J. A. (2004). "Determining the contribution of asphyxia to brain damage in the neonate." J Obstet Gynaecol Res 30(4): 276-286.

Low, J. A., A. B. Froese, et al. (1993). "The association between preterm newborn hypotension and hypoxemia and outcome during the first year." Acta Paediatr 82(5): 433-437.

Malamitsi-Puchner, A., N. Vrachnis, et al. (2006). "Investigation of midtrimester amniotic fluid factors as potential predictors of term and preterm deliveries." Mediators Inflamm 2006(4): 94381.

Martens, S. E., M. Rijken, et al. (2003). "Is hypotension a major risk factor for neurological morbidity at term age in very preterm infants?" Early Hum Dev 75(1-2): 79-89.

McDonald, J. W., M. V. Johnston, et al. (1990). "Differential ontogenic development of three receptors comprising the NMDA receptor/channel complex in the rat hippocampus." Exp Neurol 110(3): 237-247.

Meyer, U., J. Feldon, et al. (2006). "Immunological stress at the maternal-foetal interface: a link between neurodevelopment and adult psychopathology." Brain Behav Immun 20(4): 378-388.

Meyer, U., M. Nyffeler, et al. (2006). "The time of prenatal immune challenge determines the specificity of inflammation-mediated brain and behavioral pathology." J Neurosci 26(18): 4752-4762.

Mitani, A., Y. Andou, et al. (1992). "Selective vulnerability of hippocampal CA1 neurons cannot be explained in terms of an increase in glutamate concentration during ischemia in the gerbil: brain microdialysis study." Neuroscience 48(2): 307-313.

Murphy, D. J., P. L. Hope, et al. (1997). "Neonatal risk factors for cerebral palsy in very preterm babies: case-control study." BMJ 314(7078): 404-408.

Nelson, K. B., J. M. Dambrosia, et al. (1998). "Neonatal cytokines and coagulation factors in children with cerebral palsy." Ann Neurol 44(4): 665-675.

Nelson, K. B. and J. K. Grether (1995). "Can magnesium sulfate reduce the risk of cerebral palsy in very low birthweight infants?" Pediatrics 95(2): 263-269.

Palmer, C., J. Towfighi, et al. (1993). "Allopurinol administered after inducing hypoxia-ischemia reduces brain injury in 7-day-old rats." Pediatr Res 33(4 Pt 1): 405-411.

Pearce, W. (2006). "Hypoxic regulation of the fetal cerebral circulation." J Appl Physiol 100(2): 731-738.

Perlman, J. M., R. Risser, et al. (1996). "Bilateral cystic periventricular leukomalacia in the premature infant: associated risk factors." Pediatrics 97(6 Pt 1): 822-827.

Peterson, B. S., B. Vohr, et al. (2000). "Regional brain volume abnormalities and long-term cognitive outcome in preterm infants." JAMA 284(15): 1939-1947.

Pierson, C. R., R. D. Folkerth, et al. (2007). "Gray matter injury associated with periventricular leukomalacia in the premature infant." Acta Neuropathol 114(6): 619-631.

Reiter, R. J., D. X. Tan, et al. (2000). "Actions of melatonin in the reduction of oxidative stress. A review." J Biomed Sci 7(6): 444-458.

Rosin, C., T. E. Bates, et al. (2004). "Excitatory amino acid induced oligodendrocyte cell death in vitro: receptor-dependent and -independent mechanisms." J Neurochem 90(5): 1173-1185.

Rossi, D. J., T. Oshima, et al. (2000). "Glutamate release in severe brain ischaemia is mainly by reversed uptake." Nature 403(6767): 316-321.

Tan, W. K., C. E. Williams, et al. (1992). "Suppression of postischemic epileptiform activity with MK-801 improves neural outcome in fetal sheep." Ann Neurol 32(5): 677-682.

Trounce, J. Q., D. E. Shaw, et al. (1988). "Clinical risk factors and periventricular leucomalacia." Arch Dis Child 63(1): 17-22.

Volpe, J. J. (2009). "Brain injury in premature infants: a complex amalgam of destructive and developmental disturbances." Lancet Neurol 8(1): 110-124.

Vrachnis, N., N. Vitoratos, et al. (2010). "Intrauterine inflammation and preterm delivery." Ann N Y Acad Sci 1205: 118-122.

Welin, A. K., M. Sandberg, et al. (2005). "White matter injury following prolonged free radical formation in the 0.65 gestation fetal sheep brain." Pediatr Res 58(1): 100-105.

Woodward, L. J., P. J. Anderson, et al. (2006). "Neonatal MRI to predict neurodevelopmental outcomes in preterm infants." N Engl J Med 355(7): 685-694.

Wu, Y. W. (2002). "Systematic review of chorioamnionitis and cerebral palsy." Ment Retard Dev Disabil Res Rev 8(1): 25-29.

Yoon, B. H., J. K. Jun, et al. (1997). "Amniotic fluid inflammatory cytokines (interleukin-6, interleukin-1beta, and tumor necrosis factor-alpha), neonatal brain white matter lesions, and cerebral palsy." Am J Obstet Gynecol 177(1): 19-26.

Yoon, B. H., R. Romero, et al. (2000). "Fetal exposure to an intra-amniotic inflammation and the development of cerebral palsy at the age of three years." Am J Obstet Gynecol 182(3): 675-681.

Yuan, T. M., Y. Sun, et al. (2010). "Intrauterine infection/inflammation and perinatal brain damage: role of glial cells and Toll-like receptor signaling." J Neuroimmunol 229(1-2): 16-25.

Zupan, V., P. Gonzalez, et al. (1996). "Periventricular leukomalacia: risk factors revisited." Dev Med Child Neurol 38(12): 1061-1067.

5

Parenchymatous Brain Injury in Premature Infants: Intraventricular Hemorrhage and Periventricular Leukomalacia

Mauricio Barría and Ana Flández
Universidad Austral de Chile,
Hospital Clínico Regional Valdivia,
Chile

1. Introduction

Prematurity is a condition associated with high mortality and overall survived rates are near 77.5% (Stoll et al., 2010).Those who survived are at high risk of severe impairment (Bassler et al., 2009). Two percent of all live births are premature with less than 32 weeks of gestational age and 1.5% of them are very low birth weight (Mathews et al., 2011). The most common injury affecting brain of these children is periventricular leukomalacia (PVL) and intraventricular hemorrhage (IVH). PVL is the main cause of cognitive behavioural, motor and sensory impairments found in children born before 32 weeks of gestational age (Volpe, 2003). IVH has a negative impact on the neurodevelopmental outcome and is due not only to the direct consequences of IVH but also associated lesions, such as posthemorrhagic hydrocephalus (PHH) and PVL. The knowledge, prevention, diagnosis and early treatment of these clinical conditions improve the prognosis and neurological outcomes.

2. Brain injury in the premature infant

2.1 Intraventricular hemorrhage

In the late 1970s the incidence of IVH was near 50%. At the present time it is near 20 to 30%. The absolute number of infants with IVH remains significant due to increase survival rate of premature infants especially in very low birth weight, who are at high risk of IVH. Virtually all IVH in premature infants occurs within the first five days of life, with 50, 25 and 15 percent on the first, second and third day respectively, and 10 percent on the fourth day or after. IVH progresses over three to five days in approximately 20 to 40 percent of cases (Volpe, 2008; Groenendaal et al., 2010). PHH, periventricular hemorrhagic infarction (PVHI), and PVL are the most important sequelae of IVH. The first occurs in approximately 25% of infants with IVH and usually it begins within one to three weeks after the brain bleeding (Murphy et al., 2002). PVHI pathogenesis is thought to result from infarction caused by venous obstruction after a germinal matrix IVH (Bassan, 2009; Volpe, 1998). The parietal and frontal cerebral areas are the most often involved (Bassan et al., 2006a). PVL is the mayor form of brain white matter in neonates especially in premature infants. There is a strong association between PVL and IVH and data suggest the IVH may exacerbate PDL (Bassan,

2009). The short term outcome is closely related to the severity of IVH (Kusters et al., 2009). The long term outcome of infants, who survive of IVH, worsens with increasing severity of IVH and decreasing gestational age (Sherlock et al., 2005; Luu et al., 2009).

2.1.1 Risk factors and pathogenesis

IVH originates from the fragile involuting vessels of subependymal germinal matrix, located in the caudothalamic groove. The pathogenesis of this in preterm infants has been demonstrated to be related to numerous risk factors which can be divided into intravascular, probably the most important and amenable to preventive efforts, vascular and extravascular factors (Table 1). Intravascular factors are ischemia and reperfusion, like in volume infusion after hypotension, fluctuating cerebral blood flow (CBF), like in mechanical ventilation, increase in CBF, like in hypertension, anemia and hipercarbia, increase in cerebral venous pressure and platelet dysfunction and coagulation disturbances. Vascular factors consider tenuous and involuting capillaries with large diameter lumen. Extravascular factors are deficient vascular support and excessive fibrinolytic activity (Perlman et al., 1983; Lou, 1988; Pryds et al., 1989). For developing PVHI the risk factors are low birth gestational age, low Apgar scores, early life acidosis, patent ductus arteriosus, pneumothorax, pulmonary hemorrhage and needed for significant respiratory or blood pressure support (Bassan et al., 2006b). PHH likely relates at least in part to impaired cerebral spinal fluid resorption or obstruction of the acueduct or the foramina of Luschka or Magendie by particulate clot (Larroche, 1972).

Pathogenesis of IVH	
Intravascular factors	Ischemia / reperfusion Fluctuating cerebral blood flow Increase in cerebral blood flow Increase in cerebral venous pressure Platelet dysfunction and coagulation disturbances
Vascular factors	Tenous, involuting capillaries with large diameter lumen
Extravascular factors	Deficient vascular support Excessive fibrinolytic activity

Table 1. Pathogenesis of IVH.

2.1.2 Classification – Severity and grading of IVH

There are two main systems for grading the severity of IVH based on the amount of blood in the germinal matrix and lateral ventricles demonstrated by ultrasound or computed tomography (CT) scan (Table 2). By US, Volpe grades the IVH in: I, for germinal matrix hemorrhage (GMH) with no or minimal IVH, with less than 10% of ventricular volume occupying, II for IVH occupying 10%-50% of ventricular area on parasagittal view, III for IVH occupying more than 50% of ventricular area on parasagittal view, usually distends lateral ventricle. Separate notation: persistent periventricular echodensity (Volpe, 2008). Using CT scan Papile grading system is: I for isolated germinal matrix hemorrhage II for IVH without ventricular dilatation, III for IVH with ventricular dilatation and IV for IVH with parenchymal hemorrhage (Papile et al., 1978).

Reference	Method	Grading	Findings
Papile (1978)	Computed Tomography	I	Isolated germinal matrix hemorraghe (without IVH)
		II	IVH without ventricular dilatation
		III	IVH with ventricular dilatation
		IV	IVH without ventricular dilatation
Volpe (2008)	Cranial Ultrasonography	I	Germinal matrix hemorraghe with no or minimal IVH (10% ventricular volume)
		II	IVH occupying 10-50% of ventricular area
		III	IVH occupying >50% of ventricular area

Table 2. Grading IVH by Computed Tomography and Cranial Ultrasonography.

2.1.3 Clinical presentation and diagnosis

Clinical presentation varies from a silent syndrome, recognized only when a routine cranial US is performed, a mild form with decreased levels of consciousness , hypotonia, abnormal eye movements or skew deviation. A catastrophic way with rapid and severe neurological deterioration, with seizures, tonic posturing and coma is more rarely (Soul, 2008).

Whereas any cerebral imaging test is useful, it is almost invariably made by portable cranial US. The diagnosis of HIV and PHH is easy and performing fast, quick to make. Premature infants are fragile patients carry them to make CT scan or magnetic resonance adds more costs, time and risk, and there are hospitals where this exams aren´t available.

2.1.4 Prevention and treatment

The most effective strategy to prevent IVH is the prevention of preterm birth. When it cannot be avoided, the following prenatal and delivery interventions are associated with a reduced risk of IVH. Antenatal corticosteroids, reducing de risk of IVH detected by cranial US examination (OR 0.29, $CI_{95\%}$ 0.14 to 0.61) (Crowley, 2000). Delayed clamping of the umbilical cord more than 30 seconds demonstrated a lower relative risk of IVH versus early clamping (RR 0.56, $CI_{95\%}$ 0.36 to 0.93) (Rabe et al., 2004). Mothers who are at risk of preterm delivery must be transferred to a perinatal center with experience in high risk deliveries and care of prematures. Infants who are transferred after delivery are at higher risk for developing IVH. Inborn patients compared to those who are transported had a lower incidence of IVH (13.2 versus 27.4) and a lower relative distribution of severe IVH (39.2 versus 44.1 percent) (Mohamed & Aly, 2010). Delivery mode does not appear to affect the risk of severe IVH (Riskin et al., 2008) whereas the presence or absence of labor in cesarean delivery the data are conflicting. In the neonatal care units the efforts must be put on: prompt and appropriate resuscitation of the neonate, avoiding hemodynamic instability, hypoxia, hyperoxia, hypercarbia and hypocarbia. All this factors affects the cerebrovascular autoregulation; avoid hypotension and hypertension and hemodynamic instability must be care avoiding large bolus infusions. Metabolic abnormalities such hyperosmolarity, hyperglicemia and hypoglicemia should be prevented. Abnormalities in coagulation should be corrected (Bada et al., 1990; Dani et al., 2009; Perry et al., 1990).

The incidence of IVH is higher in preterm infants with patent ductus arteriosus, they should be treating (Jim et al., 2005). Ineffective interventions for prevention IVH includes: antenatal administration of phenobarbital (Shankaran et al., 1997), antenatal administration of magnesium sulfate and vitamin K to the mother has no benefit in prevent IVH (Crowther et al., 2010; Volpe, 2008). Postnatal indomethacin and vitamin E are associated a lower risk of IVH, but the first increases other risks like gastrointestinal and renal negative effects and the other with an increased risk of sepsis, so it's use is controversial (Fowlie et al., 2010; Brion et al., 2003).

The treatment doesn´t includes a specific therapy, it is supportive and the main goal is to preserve more perfectly cerebral perfusion. Treatment and early detection of complications like seizures and PHH, with serial cranial US, will improve the outcome, minimizing further brain injury.

2.1.5 Evolution and prognosis

IVH is still an important cause of injury in premature infants. The negative impact of IVH on neurodevelopmental outcome is due not only to direct consequences of IVH because it is also associated to other lesions like PHH or PVL. Long term prognosis for infants with IVH varies considerably depending on the severity of IVH, complications or other brain lesions such PVL, the most lower birth weight and gestational age add to others significant illness will determinate the outcome. Studies have suggested that preterm infants with grade I-II IVH have an increased risk of cerebral palsy and cognitive impairment compared who those without (Sherlock et al., 2005; Ancel et al., 2006; Patra et al., 2006). Infants with the mayor complications, like PVHI and PHH are at much higher risk of permanent neurologic impairments like cerebral palsy than dose with IVH alone (de Vries et al., 1999). More than 50% of children born before 32 weeks gestational age have school difficulties whether or not they had IVH, although the risk is clearly higher among children and adolescents with a story of IVH and lower birth gestational age or weight (Bowen et al., 2002; van de Bor & den Ouden, 2004). These cognitive or behavioural handicaps are related in part to white matter brain injury. The most effective strategy to prevent IVH is the prevention of preterm birth.

2.2 Periventricular leukomalacia

PVL refers to damage of cerebral white matter brain injury. The name is based on the characteristic distribution and consists of periventricular focal necrosis with subsequent cystic formation and more diffuse cerebral white matter injury (Volpe, 2008).

PVL is the mayor form of brain white matter injury that affects premature infants and it is associated with subsequent development of cerebral palsy, intellectual impairment and visual disturbances. The great risk for developing PVL is under 32 weeks of gestational age. The incidence of PVL varies among centers and in relation with imaging testing realized. Based on US, frequency of PVL ranges from 5 to 15% in VLBW infants (Stevenson et al., 1998). Using MRI, white matter abnormalities are found in 21%, and are associated with adverse neurodevelopment outcomes at a corrected age of 2 years. Gray matter abnormalities are present in half of infants, and are also significantly associated, but less strongly, with cognitive delay motor and cerebral palsy (Woodward et al., 2006). PVL is still the principal cause of this neurodevelopmental impairment (Volpe, 2003).

2.2.1 Risk factors and pathogenesis

PVL, lesion found predominantly in preterm infants, can be caused by ischemia or infection. The distinctive lesion of PVL found in the immature white matter newborns likely results from the interaction of multiple pathogenic factors (Table 3).

	Pathogenesis of PVL
Vascular anatomic factors	Incomplete development of vessels Boundary zone around the ventricles
Circulatory factors	Impaired cerebral vascular autoregulation and vasoconstriction
Cellular factors	Cystic PVL: affects all cell components Non cystic PVL: affects predominantly oligodendrocytes
Oxidative stress	Associated to: maternal/fetal infection Cytokines
Axonal development	Particularly susceptible to damage Beta amyloid precursor protein identified in swollen axons around PVL (marker of axonal damage)
Genetics	Individual genetic variations

Table 3. Pathogenesis of PVL.

To date, the several mayor factors identified are: vascular anatomic factors, pressure-passive cerebral circulation, intrinsic vulnerability of cerebral white matter of the premature neonate and infection/inflammation. The anatomy of the developing cerebral vasculature renders makes the premature infant especially vulnerable to periventricular white matter injury. The area near ventricles result in a boundary zone, with incomplete development of vessels that penetrates the deep and subcortical white matter, therefore this area is vulnerable to reduced flow (Takashima & Tanaka, 1978; Rorke, 1992).The circulatory factors and metabolic disturbances can impair autoregulation, resulting in higher risk for developing PVL, like HIV. In cystic PVL necrotic changes usually affects all cell components. Diffuse non cystic PVL affects predominantly a specific cell lineage, that of oligodendrocytes (Oka et al., 1993). Another risk factor is oxidative stress attributed to cerebral ischemia and reperfusion and or maternal infection (Khwaja & Volpe, 2008). Expression of inducible nitric oxide synthase is increased in brains with PVL (Haynes et al., 2009). Axonal maturation studies suggest that axons may be particularly susceptible to damage at time in development that coincides with the highest risk of PVL (Haynes et al., 2005). Antenatal risk factors like infection increase the risk of premature birth. In a meta-analysis, chorioamnionitis was associated with cystic PVL (RR 3.0) and cerebral palsy (RR 1.9) (Pidcock et al., 1990). Cytokines produced as a consequence of maternal or fetal infection, even the infection is asymptomatic may be associated with PVL, because the white matter is especially susceptible to damage mediated by this inflammation factor (Dammann & Leviton, 1997).

2.2.2 Classification – Severity and grading PVL

Using cranial ultrasound PVL can be classified according to Volpe or de Vries (Volpe, 1990; de Vries et al., 1992). Volpe categorizes PVL in mild, with micro cysts smaller than 0.2 mm in specially in parasagittal view, moderate with cysts between 0.2 to 0.5 mm, and severe when exists multiple cyst bilaterally bigger than 0.5 mm. According to de Vries, PVL can be classified from I to IV grades (Table 4).

Reference	Method	Grading	Findings
de Vries (1992)	Cranial Ultrasonography	I	transient periventricular echodensities persisting for ≥ 7
		II	transient periventricular echodensity evolving into small, lo-calised fronto-parietal cysts
		III	periventricular echodensities evolving into extensive periven-tricular cystic lesions
		IV	densities extending into the deep white matter evolving intoextensive cystic lesions
Volpe (1990)	Cranial Ultrasonography	Mild	micro cysts smaller than 0.2 mm
		Moderate	cysts between 0.2 to 0.5 mm
		Severe	multiples cysts bilaterally bigger than 0.5 mm

Table 4. Grading PVL by Cranial Ultrasonography.

The existence of echogenic lesions without cysts formation for more than 14 days is considered as persistent periventricular echogenicity (Larroque et al., 2003).

For RMI the grading of PVL is more descriptive. Several studies have shown that MRI is more sensitive than cranial US for detection of PVL especially for non cystic form of PVL (Maalouf et al., 2001; Roelants-van Rijn et al., 2001).

2.2.3 Diagnosis

PVL is detected in newborns by brain imaging using US or CT or RMI. Ultrasound is the initial standard method because is portable and less expensive. The criteria for US diagnosis are not well defined. A standard examination includes coronal and sagital view (Veyrac et al., 2006). The US findings evolve on repeated examinations. The cysts appear after one or three weeks and disappear after one or three months if they are moderate or severe ventriculomegaly may results (Blankenberg et al., 1997). US has limited sensitivity and specificity to detect PVL specially if the lesion are less than 0.5 cm. Sonograms may detect only one third of lesion identified at autopsy (Papile, 1997). The routine ultrasound recommended by the Quality Standard Subcommittee of the America Academy of Neurology and the Practice Committee of the Child Neurology Society made the following recommendations: Routine ultrasound screening should be performed on all infants with gestational age less than 30 weeks. Screening should be performed at 7 to 14 days of age and repeated at 36 to 40 weeks postmenstrual age. This strategy is designed to detect unsuspected PVHI, development of PHH or ventriculomegaly. CT scanning is less useful for the diagnosis of PVL in the very preterm infant because it detects fewer lesions than does MRI or US (Keeney et al., 1991). Whereas MRI is the most sensible examination the routing use of MRI scans for all premature infants has not be recommended although it may be useful in some high risk premature infants or older infant or child born prematurely who presents with cognitive, motor or sensory impairment (Ment et al., 2002).

2.2.4 Prevention and treatment

The strategies to prevent PVL emphasize the maintenance of cerebral perfusion. All conditions that impair cerebrovascular autoregulation should avoid by correcting abnormalities in blood pressure and blood gases. Antenatal exposure to betamethasone may be associated with decrease risk of cystic PVL, more than in infants whose mothers received dexamethasone or no received glucocorticoid treatment (Baud et al., 1999). Management of PDL after discharge from the hospital is directed at identification of any cognitive, sensory or motor impairments, and appropriate therapies for any such impairment. Promising studies of neuroprotective strategies to prevent or minimize PVL are being conducted in animal models, but human trials of such agents are probably still years away (Oka et al., 1993; Follett et al., 2004).

2.2.5 Evolution and prognosis

Cranial US and brain MRI may yield prognostic information in neonates and children with PVL. Infants with more extensive white matter injuries and persistent ventricular enlargements are more likely to have severe motor and cognitive deficits. When PVL and cystic formation are found in the neonatal period using US, exist a subsequent risk for developing cerebral palsy. In a twelve studies review 50% of infants with periventricular echolucency developed cerebral palsy compared with 2.6% with infants with normal cranial US scans (Holling & Leviton, 1999). Considering the increase on survival rates of extremely preterm infants (birth weight less than 1000g it would be reasonable to consider MRI to add more prognostic information for such high risk infants. Abnormal white matter a gray matter findings on brain MRI at term are predictors of adverse neurodevelopment outcome. In VLBW there is an approximately 10% incidence of cerebral palsy and up to 50%incidence of school difficulties largely due to PVL with PVHI being the other cerebral lesion that contributes significantly to neurologic disabilities. The incidence of neurologic impairments increases with lower gestational age at birth. Cerebral palsy in children born before 36 weeks gestational age is 20%. Spastic diparesis is the most common form of cerebral palsy in children born prematurely because PVL typically affects the periventricular white matter closest to the ventricles (Ancel et al., 2006). Despite of these negative numbers thanks to therapy and family support some of these children get a social adaptation that increases the quality of their lives.

3. A Chilean experience

From the years 2001 to 2006, we carried out a prospective cohort study at a tertiary care hospital at Valdivia, Chile that includes all inborn neonates with gestational age of 32 weeks or less and birth weight of 1500 g or less (Barria & Flandez, 2008). Neonates dead within first seven days of age, with major malformation at birth or transferred to another center without ultrasound evaluation were excluded. For this study an experienced pediatric neurologist performed serial cranial ultrasound to 164 neonates according the protocol of the Chilean Ministry of Health. The images were obtained by using a 7.5-MHz transducer with Medison Mysono 201® equipment. The US began within the first week of life, and then at 15 and 30 days.

The following epidemiological and clinical variables were obtained from all premature infants: gestational age, birth weight, adequacy of weight to gestational age, gender, Apgar score, antenatal use of corticosteroids, type of delivery, rupture of membranes, maternal pre-eclampsia and chorioamnionitis.

Based on the main outcome (IVH: yes/no; PVL: yes/no), variables among groups were compared using Fisher exact test for categorical data and the Student t-test or Mann-Whitney U test for continuous variables. Relative risk (RR) and its 95% confidence interval ($CI_{95\%}$) were calculated as univariate estimation of the risk of IVH and PVL. Adjusted odds ratios (OR) were estimated using multiple logistic regression with backward stepwise incorporation into the initial model of every variable showing a P value $\leq .25$ after the univariate analysis. The established level of statistical significance was $p < .05$. Data processing and analysis were carried out using Stata 8.1 (Stata Corporation, College Station, Texas).

3.1 Incidence of IVH and PVL, and factors related

The accumulated incidence of IVH was 18.3% (30/164), distributed in 30% grade I (9/30), 36.7% grade II, (11/30), 20% grade III (6/30) and 13.3% grade IV (4/30). The percentual distribution of IVH by birth weight and gestational age is show in figure 1 and 2, respectively.

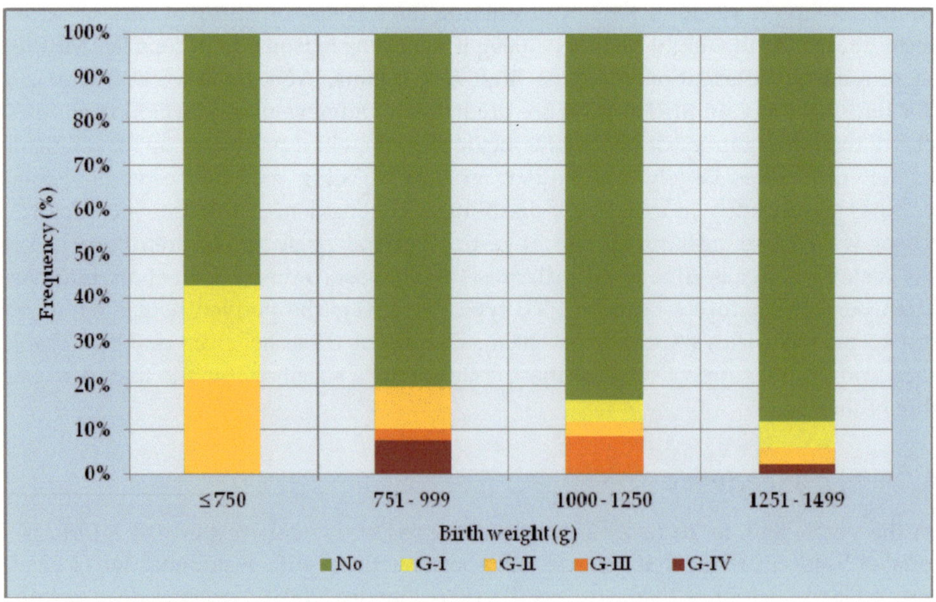

Fig. 1. Incidence of IVH by birth weight categories.

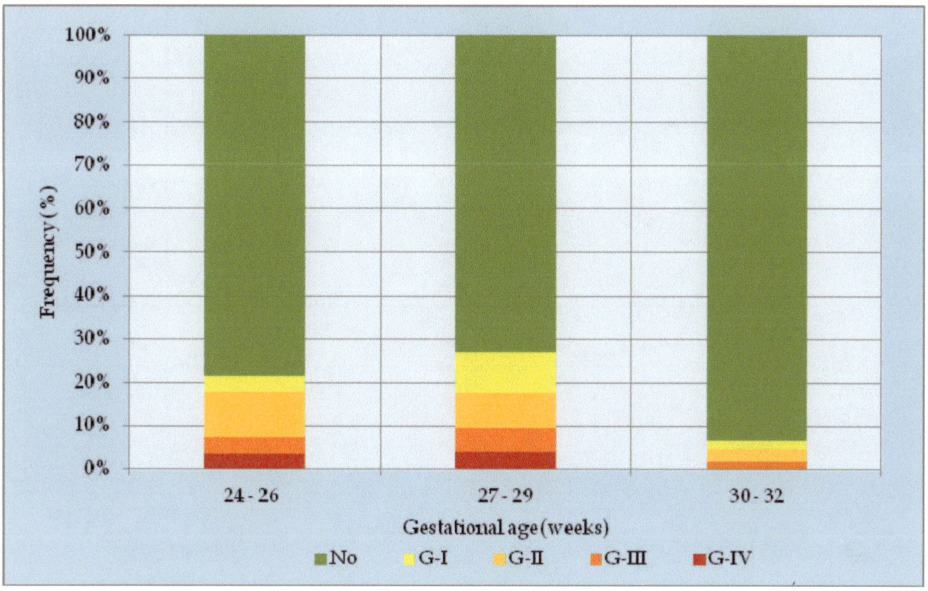

Fig. 2. Incidence of IVH by gestational age categories.

In the univariate analysis IVH was significantly associated with birth weight, estimating an OR of 5.6 ($CI_{95\%}$ 1.4 to 21.8) in infants under 750g. In other weight categories there was no significant association. According with gestational age, comparing with the group over 30 weeks, a significantly association was found in infants among 24-26 weeks (OR 5.4, $CI_{95\%}$ 1.72 to 16.7) and among 27-29 weeks (OR 5.4, $CI_{95\%}$ 1.72 to 16.7). On the other hand, the Apgar at first minute showed a significant reduction in the risk of IVH for each additional point in the score (OR 0.82, $CI_{95\%}$ 0.70 to 0.95). Other factors analyzed (chorioamnionitis, rupture of membranes, pre-eclampsia, etc.) were not significantly associated with IVH. In multivariate analysis, only Apgar at one minute was associated independently of the outcome of interest.

Ultrasound assessment allowed the detection of 61 neonates (37.2%) with abnormal white matter, 22 with PPVE and 39 with cystic lesion. Thus, the overall incidence for each event was 13.4 and 23.8% respectively. PVL was classified as mild in 64.1% (25/39), moderate in 30.8% (12/39) and severe in 5.1% (2/39). In addition, 23.3% of children with IVH also developed PVL (7/30). While PPVE was found in 50% (2/4) at 24 weeks of gestational age, a lower incidence remained relatively stable between 25 and 30 weeks, fluctuating between 14.3 and 16.7%, and declined clearly from week 31. For its part, the c-PVL was found most often below 28 weeks, accumulating 66.7% of cases (26/39). Between 24 and 27 weeks, the PVL incidence reached at least 50%, and significantly decreased from week 28 (Figure 3). A similar pattern occurred in the distribution of c-PVL and PPVE by weight strata, which the highest incidence occurred under 1000 g, reaching to below 750 g up to 21.4 and 64.3%, respectively. Additionally, the severity of periventricular lesions was higher in most premature infants, finding medians of gestational age for PPVE, mild c-PVL and moderate to severe c-PVL of 29, 27 and 26.5 weeks, respectively.

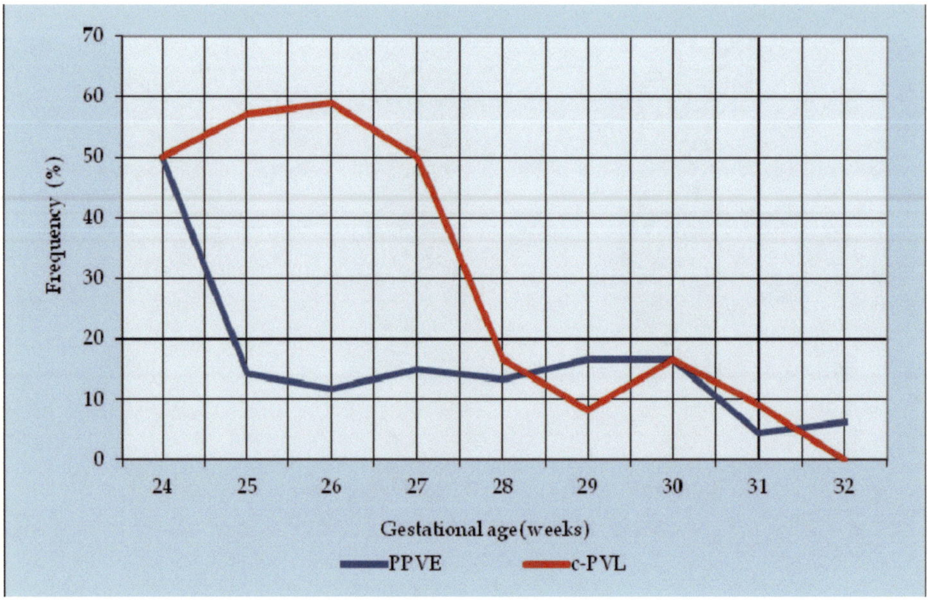

Fig. 3. Distribution of PPVE and c-PVL by gestational age.

Birth weight, gestational age, Apgar score and maternal hypertension were significantly associated with c-PVL ($p<0.05$). There were no significant differences in other characteristics assessed such as chorioamnionitis, antenatal corticosteroids nor other perinatal factors. In the univariate risk estimation, there was an increased risk of c-PVL in extremely low-birth weight newborns (<1000g) (RR 5.18, $CI_{95\%}$ 2.8 to 9.61) and in infant under 28 weeks of gestational age (RR 4.83, $CI_{95\%}$ 2.72 to 8.58). A risk reduction effect at border of statistic significance was detected for the presence of maternal hypertension (RR 0.48, $CI_{95\%}$ 0.23 to 1.02). There was no effect of Apgar score and other perinatal conditions on the development of c-PVL. To PPVE, we found an increased risk with Apgar score ≤ 3 at one minute and presence of IVH. The male showed a risk reduction in the limit of statistical significance ($p=0.058$). The extremely low-birth weight and prematurity below 28 weeks showed no association with PPVE.

Our results verify the effect of gestational age (prematurity) and birth weight commented previously in this chapter. Highlight of our findings the association found between PVL and pre-eclampsia. Consistent with this finding, a study previously has reported that children of whose mothers developed preeclampsia with intrauterine growth retardation had a low incidence of PVL (0.9%) and showed a significantly lower risk of cystic lesions (OR 0.08, CI95% 0,02 to 0.41) (Baud et al., 2000). In this sense, other study showed that none of the infants with a history of preeclampsia had c-PVL (Murata et al., 2005). However, other researchers found that this effect has been limited until 32 weeks, observing, on the contrary, an increased risk in children between 33 and 35 weeks of gestational age (Resch et al., 2000). Consequently, although the evidence is unclear, there is pathophysiologic support for considering hypertension in pregnancy as a protective factor on the incidence of c-PVL, based on self-regulatory mechanisms of the fetoplacental circulation developed in response to fluctuations of vascular tone. This would allow deal adequately potential hypoxic-ischemic episodes in the fetal brain. In this function, activation of the renin-angiotensin system in the fetoplacental unit caused by pre-eclampsia, would have a principal action (Ito et al., 2002). Likewise, hypertension and growth restriction can accelerate neurological maturity (Hadi, 1984), suggesting that early maturation may reduce brain disorders. It is also likely, however, that there are intermediate factors in this causal chain that must be clarified.

3.2 Follow up at four years

From 153 children potentially eligible born between September 2001 and June 2005 were included 81 preterm infants <32 weeks and/or VLBW with neurological evaluation at the fourth year of life (52.9%). Of the remainder, in 12 cases there was no record and in 60 there was no neurological control at this age. We calculated the incidence of neurological disorders and assessed association for different variables using t-test and Fisher exact test. Risks were calculated for overall and specific neurological areas for different variables, by estimating crude and adjusted odds ratio using multiple logistic regression.

At discharge from the hospital, 17.5% of the infants developed IVH and 23.4% cystic PVL of varying degrees. At 4 years, 30.9% of patients were diagnosed with some degree of alteration in any of the evaluated areas. Eighteen children (22.2%) showed cognitive impairment: 61% mild, 33.3% moderate and 5.5% severe. In motor area, 16 children showed affection, highlighting 37.5% (6/16) of spastic diplegia and 43.7% (7/16) hemiparesis. Six children (7.4%) showed sensory (visual, auditory or both) and social deficits.

In multivariate analysis, the gestational age was significantly associated with motor disorder estimating an adjusted OR 0.57 for each additional week ($CI_{95\%}$ 0.40 to 0.81). The history of IVH also showed a significant association estimating an OR 4.3($CI_{95\%}$ 1.1 to 17.7). Similarly, for cognitive impairment, was estimated a lower risk with higher gestational age (OR 0.64, ($CI_{95\%}$ 0.42 to 0.95).

4. Conclusion

Gestational age is an important predictor of neurologic outcomes and therefore the systematic monitoring of premature infants allows the diagnosis need to target intervention and/or rehabilitation for improving the quality of life of the child and family. Since prematures improve surviving, decreasing the adverse outcomes taking the best strategies to prevent brain injury is must necessary. Preventing the premature birth is the main goal. When it isn´t possible, knowing the pathofisiology of the brain lesions and it´s risk factors can minimizes the final results in terms of neurodevelopment. Strategies in early intervention for lower motor handicaps, specially in whose have cranial US altered is needed. Their periodic neurological evaluation for finding behavioural and cognitive impairments is needed for giving them the best expectations in their quality of live.

5. References

Ancel, P. Y., Livinec, F., Larroque, B., Marret, S., Arnaud, C., Pierrat, V. et al. (2006). Cerebral palsy among very preterm children in relation to gestational age and neonatal ultrasound abnormalities: the EPIPAGE cohort study. *Pediatrics,* Vol.117, No.3, (March 2006), pp. (828-835), ISSN 0031-4005.

Bada, H. S., Korones, S. B., Perry, E. H., Arheart, K. L., Pourcyrous, M., Runyan, J. W., III et al. (1990). Frequent handling in the neonatal intensive care unit and intraventricular hemorrhage. *The Journal of Pediatrics,* Vol.117, No.1 Pt 1, (July 1990), pp. (126-131). ISSN 0022-3476.

Barria, R. M. & Flandez, J. (2008). [Leukomalacia and periventricular echogenicity in very low birth weight premature infants]. *Revista de Neurologia,* Vol.47, No.1, (July 2008), pp. (16-20), ISSN 0210-0010.

Bassan, H. (2009). Intracranial hemorrhage in the preterm infant: understanding it, preventing it. *Clinics in Perinatology,* Vol.36, No.4, (December 2009), pp. (737-62, v), ISSN 0095-5108.

Bassan, H., Benson, C. B., Limperopoulos, C., Feldman, H. A., Ringer, S. A., Veracruz, E. et al. (2006a). Ultrasonographic features and severity scoring of periventricular hemorrhagic infarction in relation to risk factors and outcome. *Pediatrics,* Vol.117, No.6, (June 2006), pp. (2111-2118), ISSN 0031-4005.

Bassan, H., Feldman, H. A., Limperopoulos, C., Benson, C. B., Ringer, S. A., Veracruz, E. et al. (2006b). Periventricular hemorrhagic infarction: risk factors and neonatal outcome. *Pediatric Neurology,* Vol.35, No.2, (August 2006), pp. (85-92), ISSN 0887-8994.

Bassler, D., Stoll, B. J., Schmidt, B., Asztalos, E. V., Roberts, R. S., Robertson, C. M. et al. (2009). Using a count of neonatal morbidities to predict poor outcome in extremely low birth weight infants: added role of neonatal infection. *Pediatrics,* Vol.123, No.1, (January 2009), pp. (313-318), ISSN 0031-4005.

Baud, O., Foix-L'Helias, L., Kaminski, M., Audibert, F., Jarreau, P. H., Papiernik, E. et al. (1999). Antenatal glucocorticoid treatment and cystic periventricular leukomalacia in very premature infants. *The New England Journal of Medicine,* Vol.341, No.16, (October 1999), pp. (1190-1196), ISSN 0028-4793.

Baud, O., Zupan, V., Lacaze-Masmonteil, T., Audibert, F., Shojaei, T., Thebaud, B. et al. (2000). The relationships between antenatal management, the cause of delivery and neonatal outcome in a large cohort of very preterm singleton infants. *British Journal of Obstetrics and Gynaecology,* Vol.107, No.7, (July 2000), pp. (877-884), ISSN 1470-0328.

Blankenberg, F. G., Loh, N. N., Norbash, A. M., Craychee, J. A., Spielman, D. M., Person, B. L. et al. (1997). Impaired cerebrovascular autoregulation after hypoxic-ischemic injury in extremely low-birth-weight neonates: detection with power and pulsed wave Doppler US. *Radiology,* Vol.205, No.2, (November 1997), pp. (563-568), ISSN 0033-8419.

Bowen, J. R., Gibson, F. L., & Hand, P. J. (2002). Educational outcome at 8 years for children who were born extremely prematurely: a controlled study. *Journal of Paediatrics and Child Health,* Vol.38, No.5, (October 2002), pp. (438-444), ISSN 1034-4810.

Brion, L. P., Bell, E. F., & Raghuveer, T. S. (2003). Vitamin E supplementation for prevention of morbidity and mortality in preterm infants. *Cochrane Database of Systematic Reviews (Online),* No.4, CD003665, ISSN 1469-493X.

Crowley, P. (2000). Prophylactic corticosteroids for preterm birth. *Cochrane Database of Systematic Reviews (Online),* No.2, CD000065, ISSN 1469-493X.

Crowther, C. A., Crosby, D. D., & Henderson-Smart, D. J. (2010). Vitamin K prior to preterm birth for preventing neonatal periventricular haemorrhage. *Cochrane Database of Systematic Reviews (Online)*, No.1, (January 2010), CD000229, ISSN 1469-493X.

Dammann, O. & Leviton, A. (1997). Maternal intrauterine infection, cytokines, and brain damage in the preterm newborn. *Pediatric Research*, Vol.42, No.1, (July 1997), pp. (1-8), ISSN 0031-3998.

Dani, C., Poggi, C., Ceciarini, F., Bertini, G., Pratesi, S., & Rubaltelli, F. F. (2009). Coagulopathy screening and early plasma treatment for the prevention of intraventricular hemorrhage in preterm infants. *Transfusion*, Vol.49, No.12, (December 2009), pp. (2637-2644), ISSN 0041-1132.

de Vries, L. S., Eken, P., & Dubowitz, L. M. (1992). The spectrum of leukomalacia using cranial ultrasound. *Behavioural Brain Research*, Vol.49, No.1, (1992), pp. (1-6), ISSN 0166-4328.

de Vries, L. S., Groenendaal, F., van Haastert, I. C., Eken, P., Rademaker, K. J., & Meiners, L. C. (1999). Asymmetrical myelination of the posterior limb of the internal capsule in infants with periventricular haemorrhagic infarction: an early predictor of hemiplegia. *Neuropediatrics*, Vol.30, No.6, (December 1999), pp. (314-319), ISSN 0174-304X.

Follett, P. L., Deng, W., Dai, W., Talos, D. M., Massillon, L. J., Rosenberg, P. A. et al. (2004). Glutamate receptor-mediated oligodendrocyte toxicity in periventricular leukomalacia: a protective role for topiramate. *The Journal of Neuroscience*, Vol.24, No.18, (May 2004), pp. (4412-4420), ISSN 0270-6474.

Fowlie, P. W., Davis, P. G., & McGuire, W. (2010). Prophylactic intravenous indomethacin for preventing mortality and morbidity in preterm infants. *Cochrane Database of Systematic Reviews (Online)*, No.7, (July 2010), CD000174, 1469-493X.

Groenendaal, F., Termote, J. U., Heide-Jalving, M., van Haastert, I. C., & de Vries, L. S. (2010). Complications affecting preterm neonates from 1991 to 2006: what have we gained? *Acta Paediatrica*, Vol.99, No.3, (March 2010), pp. (354-358), ISSN 0803-5253.

Hadi, H. A. (1984). Fetal cerebral maturation in hypertensive disorders of pregnancy. *Obstetrics and Gynecology*, Vol.63, No.2, (February 1984), pp. (214-219), ISSN 0029-7844.

Haynes, R. L., Borenstein, N. S., Desilva, T. M., Folkerth, R. D., Liu, L. G., Volpe, J. J. et al. (2005). Axonal development in the cerebral white matter of the human fetus and infant. *The Journal of comparative Neurology*, Vol.484, No.2, (April 2005), pp. (156-167), ISSN 0021-9967.

Haynes, R. L., Folkerth, R. D., Trachtenberg, F. L., Volpe, J. J., & Kinney, H. C. (2009). Nitrosative stress and inducible nitric oxide synthase expression in periventricular leukomalacia. *Acta neuropathologica*, Vol.118, No.3, (September 2009), pp. (391-399), ISSN 0001-6322.

Holling, E. E. & Leviton, A. (1999). Characteristics of cranial ultrasound white-matter echolucencies that predict disability: a review. *Developmental Medicine and Child Neurology*, Vol.41, No.2, (February 1999), pp. (136-139), ISNN 0012-1622.

Ito, M., Itakura, A., Ohno, Y., Nomura, M., Senga, T., Nagasaka, T. et al. (2002). Possible activation of the renin-angiotensin system in the feto-placental unit in preeclampsia. *The Journal of Clinical Endocrinology and Metabolism*, Vol.87, No.4, (April 2002), pp. (1871-1878), ISSN 0021-972X.

Jim, W. T., Chiu, N. C., Chen, M. R., Hung, H. Y., Kao, H. A., Hsu, C. H. et al. (2005). Cerebral hemodynamic change and intraventricular hemorrhage in very low birth weight infants with patent ductus arteriosus. *Ultrasound in Medicine & Biology,* Vol.31, No.2, (February 2005), pp. (197-202), ISSN 0301-5629.

Keeney, S. E., Adcock, E. W., & McArdle, C. B. (1991). Prospective observations of 100 high-risk neonates by high-field (1.5 Tesla) magnetic resonance imaging of the central nervous system. II. Lesions associated with hypoxic-ischemic encephalopathy. *Pediatrics,* Vol.87, No.4, (April 1991), pp. (431-438), ISSN 0031-4005.

Khwaja, O. & Volpe, J. J. (2008). Pathogenesis of cerebral white matter injury of prematurity. *Archives of Disease in Childhood. Fetal and Neonatal Edition,* Vol.93, No.2, (March 2008), pp. (F153-F161), ISSN 1359-2998.

Kusters, C. D., Chen, M. L., Follett, P. L., & Dammann, O. (2009). "Intraventricular" hemorrhage and cystic periventricular leukomalacia in preterm infants: how are they related? *Journal of Child Neurology,* Vol.24, No.9, (September 2009), pp. (1158-1170), ISSN 0883-0738.

Larroche, J. C. (1972). Post-haemorrhagic hydrocephalus in infancy. Anatomical study. *Biology of the Neonate,* Vol.20, No.3, pp. (287-299). ISSN 0006-3126.

Larroque, B., Marret, S., Ancel, P. Y., Arnaud, C., Marpeau, L., Supernant, K. et al. (2003). White matter damage and intraventricular hemorrhage in very preterm infants: the EPIPAGE study. *The Journal of Pediatrics,* Vol.143, No.4, (October 2003), pp. (477-483), ISSN 0022-3476.

Lou, H. C. (1988). The "lost autoregulation hypothesis" and brain lesions in the newborn--an update. *Brain & Development,* Vol.10, No.3, (1988), pp. (143-146), ISSN 0387-7604.

Luu, T. M., Ment, L. R., Schneider, K. C., Katz, K. H., Allan, W. C., & Vohr, B. R. (2009). Lasting effects of preterm birth and neonatal brain hemorrhage at 12 years of age. *Pediatrics,* Vol.123, No.3, (March 2009), pp. (1037-1044), ISSN 0031-4005.

Maalouf, E. F., Duggan, P. J., Counsell, S. J., Rutherford, M. A., Cowan, F., Azzopardi, D. et al. (2001). Comparison of findings on cranial ultrasound and magnetic resonance imaging in preterm infants. *Pediatrics,* Vol.107, No.4, (April 2001), pp. (719-727), ISSN 0031-4005.

Mathews, T. J., Minino, A. M., Osterman, M. J., Strobino, D. M., & Guyer, B. (2011). Annual summary of vital statistics: 2008. *Pediatrics,* Vol.127, No.1, (January 2011), pp. (146-157), ISSN 0031-4005.

Ment, L. R., Bada, H. S., Barnes, P., Grant, P. E., Hirtz, D., Papile, L. A. et al. (2002). Practice parameter: neuroimaging of the neonate: report of the Quality Standards Subcommittee of the American Academy of Neurology and the Practice Committee of the Child Neurology Society. *Neurology,* Vol.58, No.12, (June 2002), pp. (1726-1738), ISSN 0028-3878.

Mohamed, M. A. & Aly, H. (2010). Transport of premature infants is associated with increased risk for intraventricular haemorrhage. *Archives of Disease in Childhood. Fetal and Neonatal Edition,* Vol.95, No.6, (November 2010), pp. F403-F407, ISSN 1359-2998.

Murata, Y., Itakura, A., Matsuzawa, K., Okumura, A., Wakai, K., & Mizutani, S. (2005). Possible antenatal and perinatal related factors in development of cystic periventricular leukomalacia. *Brain & Development,* Vol.27, No.1, (January 2005), pp. (17-21), ISSN 0387-7604.

Murphy, B. P., Inder, T. E., Rooks, V., Taylor, G. A., Anderson, N. J., Mogridge, N. et al. (2002). Posthaemorrhagic ventricular dilatation in the premature infant: natural history and predictors of outcome. *Archives of Disease in Childhood. Fetal and Neonatal Edition, Vol.87,* No.1, (July 2002), pp. F37-F41, ISSN 1359-2998.

Oka, A., Belliveau, M. J., Rosenberg, P. A., & Volpe, J. J. (1993). Vulnerability of oligodendroglia to glutamate: pharmacology, mechanisms, and prevention. *The Journal of Neuroscience,* Vol.13, No.4, (April 1993), pp. (1441-1453), ISSN 0270-6474.

Papile, L. A. (1997). Intracranial hemoraghe. In: *Neonatal-Perinatal Medicine. Diseases of the Fetus and Infant,* Fanaroff,A.A. & Martin, R. J. (Eds.), Mosby year Book, ISBN 978-0-323-06545-0, St. Louis.

Papile, L. A., Burstein, J., Burstein, R., & Koffler, H. (1978). Incidence and evolution of subependymal and intraventricular hemorrhage: a study of infants with birth weights less than 1,500 gm. *The Journal of Pediatrics,* Vol.92, No.4, (April 1978), pp. (529-534), ISSN 0022-3476.

Patra, K., Wilson-Costello, D., Taylor, H. G., Mercuri-Minich, N., & Hack, M. (2006). Grades I-II intraventricular hemorrhage in extremely low birth weight infants: effects on neurodevelopment. *The Journal of Pediatrics,* Vol.149, No.2, (August 2006), pp. (169-173), ISSN 0022-3476.

Perlman, J. M., McMenamin, J. B., & Volpe, J. J. (1983). Fluctuating cerebral blood-flow velocity in respiratory-distress syndrome. Relation to the development of intraventricular hemorrhage. *The New England Journal of Medicine,* Vol.309, No.4, (July 1983), pp. (204-209), ISSN 0028-4793.

Perry, E. H., Bada, H. S., Ray, J. D., Korones, S. B., Arheart, K., & Magill, H. L. (1990). Blood pressure increases, birth weight-dependent stability boundary, and intraventricular hemorrhage. *Pediatrics,* Vol.85, No.5, (May 1990), pp. (727-732), ISSN 0031-4005.

Pidcock, F. S., Graziani, L. J., Stanley, C., Mitchell, D. G., & Merton, D. (1990). Neurosonographic features of periventricular echodensities associated with cerebral palsy in preterm infants. *The Journal of Pediatrics,* Vol.116, No.3, (March 1990), pp. (417-422), ISSN 0022-3476.

Pryds, O., Greisen, G., Lou, H., & Friis-Hansen, B. (1989). Heterogeneity of cerebral vasoreactivity in preterm infants supported by mechanical ventilation. *The Journal of Pediatrics,* Vol.115, No.4, (October 1989), pp. (638-645), ISSN 0022-3476.

Rabe, H., Reynolds, G., & Diaz-Rossello, J. (2004). Early versus delayed umbilical cord clamping in preterm infants. *Cochrane Database of Systematic Reviews (Online),* No.4, (October 2004), CD003248, ISSN 1469-493X.

Resch, B., Vollaard, E., Maurer, U., Haas, J., Rosegger, H., & Muller, W. (2000). Risk factors and determinants of neurodevelopmental outcome in cystic periventricular leucomalacia. *European Journal of Pediatrics,* Vol.159, No.9, (September 2000), pp. (663-670), ISSN 0340-6199.

Riskin, A., Riskin-Mashiah, S., Bader, D., Kugelman, A., Lerner-Geva, L., Boyko, V. et al. (2008). Delivery mode and severe intraventricular hemorrhage in single, very low birth weight, vertex infants. *Obstetrics and Gynecology,* Vol.112, No.1, (July 2008), pp. (21-28), ISSN 0029-7844.

Roelants-van Rijn, A. M., Groenendaal, F., Beek, F. J., Eken, P., van Haastert, I. C., & de Vries, L. S. (2001). Parenchymal brain injury in the preterm infant: comparison of cranial ultrasound, MRI and neurodevelopmental outcome. *Neuropediatrics,* Vol.32, No.2, (April 2001), pp. (80-89), ISSN 0174-304X.

Rorke, L. B. (1992). Anatomical features of the developing brain implicated in pathogenesis of hypoxic-ischemic injury. *Brain Pathology,* Vol.2, No.3, (July 1992), pp. (211-221), ISSN 1015-6305.

Shankaran, S., Papile, L. A., Wright, L. L., Ehrenkranz, R. A., Mele, L., Lemons, J. A. et al. (1997). The effect of antenatal phenobarbital therapy on neonatal intracranial hemorrhage in preterm infants. *The New England Journal of Medicine,* Vol.337, No.7, (August 1997), pp. (466-471), ISSN 0028-4793.

Sherlock, R. L., Anderson, P. J., & Doyle, L. W. (2005). Neurodevelopmental sequelae of intraventricular haemorrhage at 8 years of age in a regional cohort of ELBW/very preterm infants. *Early Human Development,* Vol.81, No.11, (November 2005), pp. (909-916), ISSN 0378-3782.

Soul, J. (2008). Intracranial Hemorrhage and Periventricular Leukomalacia. In: *Manual of Neonatal Care,*Cloherty,J.P., Eichenwald, E. C., & Stark, A. R. (Eds.), pp. (500-518), Lippincott Williams & Wilkins, ISBN 978-0-7817-6984-6, Philadelphia, USA.

Stevenson, D. K., Wright, L. L., Lemons, J. A., Oh, W., Korones, S. B., Papile, L. A. et al. (1998). Very low birth weight outcomes of the National Institute of Child Health and Human Development Neonatal Research Network, January 1993 through December 1994. *American Journal of Obstetrics and Gynecology,* Vol.179, No.6 Pt 1, (December1998), pp. (1632-1639), ISSN 0002-9378.

Stoll, B. J., Hansen, N. I., Bell, E. F., Shankaran, S., Laptook, A. R., Walsh, M. C. et al. (2010). Neonatal outcomes of extremely preterm infants from the NICHD Neonatal Research Network. *Pediatrics,* Vol.126, No.3, (September 2010), pp. (443-456), ISSN 0031-4005.

Takashima, S. & Tanaka, K. (1978). Development of cerebrovascular architecture and its relationship to periventricular leukomalacia. *Archives of Neurology, Vol.35,* No.1, (January 1978), pp. (11-16), ISSN 0003-9942.

van de Bor, M. & den Ouden, L. (2004). School performance in adolescents with and without periventricular-intraventricular hemorrhage in the neonatal period. *Seminars in perinatology,* Vol.28, No.4, (August 2004), pp. (295-303), ISSN 0146-0005.

Veyrac, C., Couture, A., Saguintaah, M., & Baud, C. (2006). Brain ultrasonography in the premature infant. *Pediatric Radiology,* Vol.36, No.7, (July 2006), pp. (626-635), ISSN 0301-0449.

Volpe, J. J. (1990). Brain injury in the premature infant: is it preventable? *Pediatric research,* Vol.27, No.6 Suppl, pp. S28-S33, ISSN 0031-3998.

Volpe, J. J. (1998). Neurologic outcome of prematurity. *Archives of Neurology,* Vol.55, No.3, (March 1998), pp. (297-300), ISSN 0003-9942.

Volpe, J. J. (2003). Cerebral white matter injury of the premature infant-more common than you think. *Pediatrics,* Vol.112, No.1 Pt 1, (July 2003), pp. (176-180), ISSN 0031-4005.

Volpe, J. J. (2008). Intracranial Hemorrhage: Germinal matrix-intraventricular hemorrhage of the premature infant. In: *Neurology of the newborn,*Volpe,J.J. (Ed.), pp. (517-588), Saunders, ISBN 1-4160-3995-3, Philadelphia, USA.

Woodward, L. J., Anderson, P. J., Austin, N. C., Howard, K., & Inder, T. E. (2006). Neonatal MRI to predict neurodevelopmental outcomes in preterm infants. *The New England Journal of Medicine,* Vol.355, No.7, (August 2006), pp. (685-694), ISSN 0028-4793.

6

Association of Meconium Stained Amniotic Fluid with Fetal and Neonatal Brain Injury

Zoe Iliodromiti[1], Charalampos Grigoriadis[2], Nikolaos Vrachnis[2], Charalampos Siristatidis[3], Michail Varras[4] and Georgios Creatsas[2]
[1]*Neonatal Unit, 2nd Department of Obstetrics and Gynecology, University of Athens Medical School, Aretaieio Hospital, Athens,*
[2]*2nd Department of Obstetrics and Gynecology, University of Athens Medical School, Aretaieio Hospital, Athens,*
[3]*3nd Department of Obstetrics and Gynecology, University of Athens Medical School, Attiko Hospital, Athens,*
[4]*Department of Obstetrics and Gynecology, Elena Hospital, Athens, Greece*

1. Introduction

Meconium stained amniotic fluid (MSAF), which occurs in about 10-15% of all pregnancies [Wiswell TE. et al., 1990], is common in term births and especially in post-date deliveries. The etiology and pathophysiology of MSAF is poorly understood. While the more advanced maturation process of the gastrointestinal tract may account for the higher rates of MSAF in post-date deliveries, it is generally believed that the presence of MSAF in other circumstances is a marker of fetal distress and may be associated with adverse fetal and neonatal outcome [Woods JR. et al., 1994; Krebs HB. et al., 1980; Mazor M. et al., 1998].

A relationship of MSAF with stillborn infants, abnormal fetal heart-rate (FHR) tracings, neonatal encephalopathy, respiratory distress (meconium aspiration syndrome, MAS) and abnormal neurologic outcome is reported in the literature. The finding of MSAF is associated with multiple markers of fetal distress, as meconium-stained infants have in general lower scalp pHs and lower umbilical cord artery pHs in comparison with infants born through clear amniotic fluid [Nathan L. et al., 1994; Ramin K. et al., 1994; Starks GD., 1980]. Additionally, infants born through MSAF have lower Apgar scores in the first and fifth minute after delivery [Wiswell TE. et al., 1990; Clifford SH., 1945]. However, in the vast majority of cases, no major problems occur in infants born through MSAF.

The term "meconium aspiration syndrome (MAS)" describes neonates born through MSAF, who present respiratory distress which cannot be otherwise explained. MAS is the most frequent complication diagnosed among infants born through MSAF, with an incidence of about 5% in these cases [Wiswell TE. et al., 1993; Cleary GM. et al., 1998]. Meconium stained infants are considered 100 times more likely to develop MAS, compared with infants born through clear amniotic fluid [Fleischer A., et al., 1992]. The severity of this syndrome is demonstrated by the fact that published data report that about one-third to one-half of neonates with MAS will require mechanical ventilation, one-quarter will develop pneumothoraxes and one in twenty will die, although the death rate has declined appreciably since the 1990s as a result of successful airway management in the delivery room, better ventilatory techniques and improvement in supportive neonatal care (thermoregulation, parenteral nutrition) [Wiswell TE. et al., 1993; Cleary GM. et al., 1998].

It is noteworthy that the significantly higher rates of admission to newborn intensive care units for neonates born through MSAF in comparison with those born through clear amniotic fluid underlines the strong association between MSAF and fetal distress; the greater experience, moreover, gained in this area has also yielded useful data about the cost-effective management of such cases. It was estimated that approximately 24% of meconium stained neonates were admitted to newborn intensive care units, compared to 7% of those born through clear amniotic fluid [Nathan L. et al., 1994].

Although the incidence of MSAF and MAS is high, there remains a distinct paucity of literature describing the neurological development of either children born through MSAF or those with MAS. The aim of this Chapter is to review studies which examine the potential association of MSAF and MAS with fetal and neonatal brain injury in order to investigate the incidence of this condition, the possible pathogenetic pathways of fetal brain injury in MSAF and the optimal means of recognizing and preventing these complications.

1.1 Historical aspects

It was the famous ancient Greek philosopher Aristotle who, first describing meconium stained amniotic fluid, conferred on this condition the name "meconium-arion", literally meaning "opium-like". His use of this term may have been due to his belief that MSAF induced fetal sleep and his knowledge that it was also associated with fetal deaths and neonatal depression, or else it may have arisen because meconium resembles the black, tarry consistency of processed opium. Several publications from the 1600s reported MSAF as a sign of death or impending death of the fetus. The first description of in utero aspiration of meconium and MAS was published in 1918 [Reed CB., 1918]. An explanation for the pathogenetic mechanism was based on the hypothesis that in utero anoxia could relax the anal sphincter and result in meconium passage. Other investigators maintained that asphyxia leads to meconium passage because of increased intestinal peristalsis [Brews A., 1948]. The critical point of hypoxia that is needed for meconium passage was first described in a study which found that umbilical venous oxygen saturation levels below 30% were associated with meconium passage [Walker J., 1954]. In 1945, Clifford, in a research study supporting the need for resuscitation in such cases and basing his views on the complications observed in neonates, reported a mortality rate of approximately 6% and a morbidity rate of about 60% among infants born through MSAF [Steer PJ. et al., 1989].

Useful conclusions with regard to MSAF and MAS were disclosed in the National Institute of Neurological and Communicative Disorders and Stroke Collaborative Perinatal Project (CPP) of the late 1950s and 1960s. In this project, more than 42,000 children were followed as from delivery for possible future identification of cerebral palsy (CP), mental retardation (MR) and other abnormal neurologic findings. It was found that 10.3% of all live-born infants in the CPP had had meconium staining. Neonatal mortality rate for the stained group was about 3.3%, compared to 1.7% among infants born through clear amniotic fluid

[Fujikura T., et al., 1975]. The incidence of MAS among infants born through MSAF in the CPP was about 8.7% [Naeye RL., 1992]. In contrast with the extremely decreased mortality rates of this complication in the present day, it was noted that ultimately 63% of neonates who developed MAS in the CPP died. It is notable that from 1957, the hypothesis that meconium stained neonates had a significantly higher risk of developing neurologic disorders in the future was supported in the literature [Brown CA. et al., 1957].

The greatly improved results in mortality and morbidity rates today in cases of infants diagnosed with MAS are attributable to the highly successfully applied aggressive airway management that has been followed by pediatricians in meconium stained neonates since the 1970s [Wiswell TE., et al., 2000]. Although large randomized controlled clinical trials do not support the need for intratracheal intubation and suctioning, the generally followed practice of obstetrical oro- and nasopharyngeal suctioning and postpartum intratracheal suctioning of meconium stained infants in the delivery room plays an important role in prevention of severe complications arising from the meconium aspiration syndrome [Wiswell TE., et al., 2000]. On the other hand, maneuvers like intrapartum oro- and nasopharyngeal suctioning prior to delivery of the baby's shoulders or amnioinfusion of normal saline or lactated Ringer's infusion into the uteri of women with MSAF do not avert the development of MAS [Vain NE. et al., 2004; Fraser WD. et al., 2004].

2. Mechanisms of meconium passage

Meconium is a viscous green liquid consisting of gastrointestinal secretions, bile, bile acids, mucus, pancreatic juice, cellular debris, amniotic fluid and swallowed vernix caseosa, lanugo and blood [Wiswell TE. et al., 1993]. Approximately 60-200 gr. of meconium are found in a term infant's intestine. The many possible pathophysiological pathways of intraamniotic meconium passage all have the same origin, which is ante- or intrapartum asphyxia. Several investigators have argued that in utero anoxia could relax the anal sphincter tone of the embryo [Reed CB., 1918], while others have expressed the hypothesis that anoxia could increase intestinal peristalsis [Brews A., 1948]. In any case, both these pathways originate from asphyxia and lead to intraamniotic meconium passage. Additionally, the theory of compression of the fetal head or umbilical cord which produces a vagal response and finally leads to meconium passage is supported in the published literature [Miller FC. et al., 1981]. The important role of hypoxia was well documented after clinical observations that umbilical venous oxygen saturation levels below 30% were associated with meconium passage [Walker J. et al., 1954]. There are also theories which propose a potential pathogenetic role of intrauterine infection leading to meconium passage, as the rate of intraamniotic infection is shown to be significantly higher in women with MSAF [Wen TW. et al., 1993; Vrachnis N. et al., 2010].

On the other hand, in the majority of cases, the presence of meconium is probably a physiologic maturational event. Meconium passage is rare before the 37th week of gestation, but may occur in more than 35% of pregnancies after the 42nd week of gestation [Nathan L. et al., 1994].

However, how can one make estimates of the amount of time that has passed between fetal defecation and birth? There are clear-cut indications. Freshly passed meconium is a thick, viscous shimmering black-green colored substance. With the progress of time, the color of

MSAF will change to brown and finally to tan or yellow. That is why the yellow-colored appearance of MSAF is synonymous with the term "old" meconium.

Additionally, it is generally believed that the duration between defecation and delivery can be estimated by the color of placental staining. Acute staining is slimy with a dark-green color, chronic staining has a characteristic muddy-brown appearance (over six hours of exposure), while very remotely passed meconium is light tan.

3. MSAF and brain injury

3.1 MSAF and adverse neurodevelopmental outcomes

Although large prospective epidemiologic studies specifically following a group of neonates born through MSAF for future development of neurologic handicaps are absent from the published literature, there are several reports which link the pathogenetic role of meconium passage with a variety of neurolodevelopmental disorders.

A strong relationship between MSAF and symptoms like hypotonia, lethargy and seizures in infants born through MSAF is documented in the literature [Brown CA. et al., 1957]. Additionally, Grafe studied cases of brain injury in 83 stillborns and 13 infants that occurred within one hour from delivery [Grafe MR., 1994]. A higher rate of neurological complications was noted among infants born through MSAF if meconium staining of the placenta was present, while the major neurologic pathological finding was white-manner gliosis or necrosis. The key role of placental meconium staining was also observed in a recent study published in 2005 which stated that meconium-associated vascular necrosis of the placenta is the main etiological factor associated with neurologic impairment in infants [Redline RW., 2005] (Figure 1).

Research studies have also recognized a strong relationship of meconium passage with adverse neurologic outcome, especially in premature labor. Meconium in premature labor is considered to be a higher risk factor for future neurologic disorders compared to term delivery. In a study of Kalis et al., 41% of premature infants born through MSAF were diagnosed as having cerebral palsy (CP), compared to 10% in the same group with clear amniotic fluid. The incidence of CP in term pregnancy when meconium was present was reported as 0.4%, compared to 0.3% in a population without any obstretical risk [Kalis V. et al., 2001].

Information and data from the CPP were examined by several investigators in order to exclude safe conclusions. A group of 50 children from the CPP diagnosed with neurological disorders, like moderate or severe motor disability and severe MR, was studied and compared to a large control population. Those with severe disorders were more than twice as likely to have been born through MSAF (40.8% vs 19.1%) [Nelson KB. et al., 1977]. The same investigator found that the rate of CP among children with a birthweight over 2500 gr. was about 3/1000 if there was no history of obstetrical problems, while it was 4/1000 when neonates were born through MSAF in the absence of further obstetrical complications [Nelson KB., 1989]. Of particular interest was the increased CP rate (94/1000) when there was a history of MSAF and a 5-minute Apgar score below 3 [Nelson KB., 1989]. In cases of neonates with a birthweight below 2500 gr. born through MSAF, the estimated rate of CP was approximately 15/1000. Additionally, 12/1000 of these low-birthweight meconium stained infants developed seizures in the absence of CP [Nelson KB. et al., 1984].

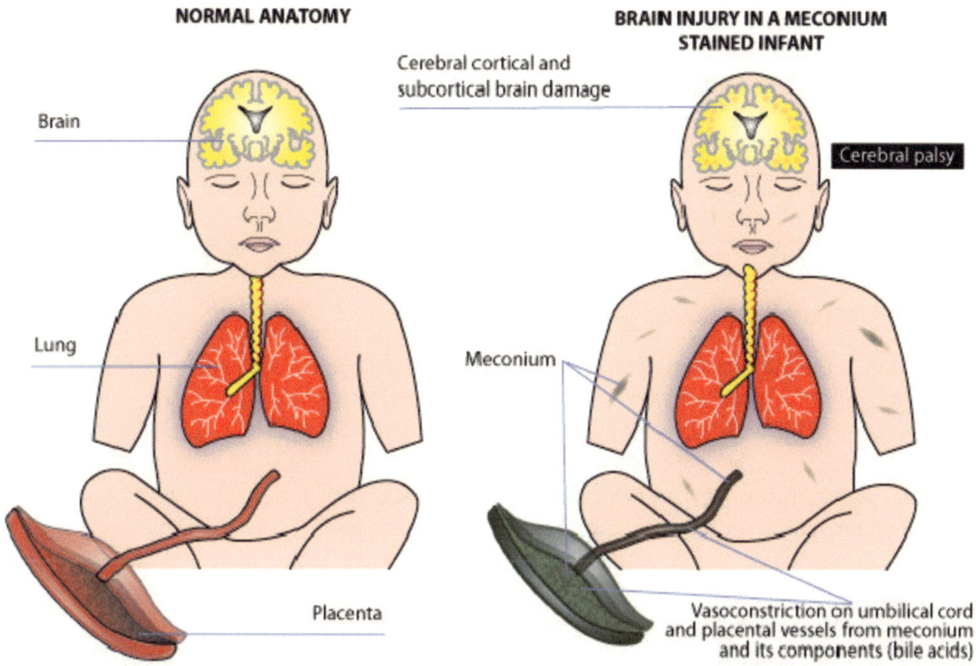

Fig. 1. Pathogenetic pathway of direct in vivo vasoconstriction on umbilical cord and placental vessels from meconium (meconium stained placenta), that leads to cerebral cortical and subcortical brain damage, in comparison with normal neural development in an infant born through clear amniotic fluid without placenta lesions (infracts or vasoconstriction).

In another study, a group of 75 babies diagnosed with CP was analyzed [Shields JR. et al., 1988]. The aim of this research was to investigate the potential correlation between MSAF/MAS and future development of CP. The results supported this hypothesis, as 41% of babies with CP had been born through MSAF, while 21% had been affected by MAS. Similar results were reported in several other studies that found an increased rate of CP and periventricular leukomalacia (PVL) among meconium stained premature infants [Gaffney G. et al., 1994; Spinillo A. et al., 1997; Spinillo A. et al., 1998].

An interesting research studied the incidence of autistic disorder in neonatal intensive care unit survivors. Five thousand two hundred seventy-one (5271) children were followed for neurodevelopmental disorders for a five-year period after discharge. Autistic disorder was diagnosed in 18 cases, while 57 developed CP. Obstetrical history of MAS was found significantly higher in the group with autistic disorder (22%) or CP (8.8%), compared with the control population of neonatal care units survivors without MAS [Matsuishi T. et al., 1999].

Several studies have also found an increased rate (up to sevenfold) of seizures during the neonatal period among infants born through MSAF in comparison with cases in which amniotic fluid was clear [Nathan L. et al., 1994; Berkus MD. et al., 1994; Sato S. et al., 2003]. This observation is important as seizures constitute a predictive factor of subsequent neurological adverse outcome. In some of these cases of seizures during the neonatal period, even in the absence of signs of hypoxic-ischemic encephalopathy, perisagittal cerebral infracts were present [Sato S. et al., 2003]. A hypothesis that pre-existing neurological injury prior to delivery takes place in the majority of meconium stained infants, rather than intrapartum injury, was supported by a recent research [Blackwell SC. et al., 2001]. In this study, the risk for developing seizures among neonates with severe MAS was found to be independent from pH levels of the umbilical cord artery, which are associated with intrapartum fetal distress. According to these findings, the conclusion that non-hypoxic-ischemic mechanisms may also cause fetal and neonatal brain injury seems correct.

3.2 MSAF and pathogenesis of brain injury

Thus, which is the pathogenetic mechanism that leads to brain injury in cases of infants born through MSAF? The pathophysiologic mechanisms that cause CP remain controversial and cannot be associated with birth injury or intrapartum hypoxic-ischemic insults alone [Kuban KCK et al., 1994]. At the present time, several markers are used for prognostic purposes, with fetal heart rate tracing, the Apgar score in the first and fifth minute after delivery or the presence of recurrent neonatal seizures providing means to indicate the potential for CP in the future. In particular, the latter prognostic factor seems to have greater validity than other perinatal characteristics [Nelson KB. et al., 1977; Kuban KCK et al., 1994]. Of course, ultrasonographic appearance of periventricular leukomalacia is the most reliable sign of future CP development [Kalis V. et al., 2001]. Nevertheless, none of these markers explains the pathogenesis of brain injury after meconium passage, since they are considered to be the consequence rather than the cause of the processes leading to CP.

In order to investigate the potential pathogenetic mechanism of fetal and neonatal brain injury due to MSAF it is necessary to emphasize the possible conditions that lead to meconium passage in utero, these conditions being: hypoxia-anoxia status, intrauterine infection or maturation progress. Consequently, meconium staining is strongly correlated with disorders that could affect the fetus: chorioamnionitis, premature rupture of membranes, abruption placentae and large placental infarcts [Naeye RL., 1992]. Some fetuses suffer acute or chronic episodes, severe enough to cause brain injury, but not intrauterine death. If the stress disappears, the fetus can resume its normal status and not present postpartum depression with low Apgar scores or low umbilical cord artery pH. The neonate may seem neurologically healthy for months after delivery; however, severe neurodevelopmental disorders could be diagnosed years after birth. Similarly, the presence of negative prognostic factors, such as abnormal fetal heart rate tracing or low Apgar scores, may reflect an insult that took place long before delivery (hours to days to even weeks or months) rather than of more immediate intrapartum difficulties.

These observations lead to the conclusion that the intrauterine environment and the causes giving rise to intraamniotic meconium passage are also involved in the pathophysiology of fetal brain injury due to MSAF. It is clear that meconium passage could be a major factor in the pathogenesis of neurological disorders.

The main pathogenetic pathways are two:

i. Meconium and its components (bile acids) may have a direct vasoconstrictive effect on umbilical and placental vessels [Kalis V. et al., 2001] (Figure 1). This hypothesis was

studied in a research seeking to investigate a potential mechanism of fetal ischemia caused by vasoconstriction of placental or umbilical vessels [Altshuler G. et al., 1989; Altshuler G., 1995]. Vasoactive substances of meconium could cross into the fetal circulation and cause ischemia of cerebral vessels or render pulmonary vessels more reactive, resulting in persistent pulmonary hypertension of the newborn. Additionally, an in vitro experiment that was performed exposing excised umbilical venous tissue to meconium showed substantial vasoconstriction. Although the specific constituent was not identified, the hypothesis that MSAF could cause in vivo placental and umbilical cord vasoconstriction was correct, as the agent was found to be heat-labile.
This pathogenetic pathway underlines the major role of meconium-induced placental necrosis, due to vasoconstrictive effects on umbilical and placental vessels, in fetal brain injury. Meconium in the amniotic fluid may sometimes initiate vasoconstriction on umbilical and placental vessels, which leads to cerebral cortical and subcortical brain damage and finally ischemic-hypoxemic CP, as it may reduce the venous return of oxygenated blood from the placenta to the fetus [Naeye RL., 1995]. This theory is in agreement with previously mentioned studies which report that a higher rate of neurological complications is noted among infants born through MSAF if meconium staining of the placenta was present, as meconium-associated vascular necrosis of the placenta is thought to be the main etiological factor associated with neurologic impairment in infants [Redline RW., 2005]. As established by Altshuler, with the passage of meconium into the fetal sac, it takes a minimum of four to twelve hours for the meconium to diffuse to and into the lumens of placental and umbilical cord vessels and become pathogenetic, inducing vasoconstriction [Altshuler G., 1995].

ii. Meconium causes intraamniotic infection and results in a release of fetal cytokines and eicosanoids (tumor necrosis factor alpha-TNF-a-, interleukin 1 beta-IL-1β-, interleukin 6 -IL-6-, interleukin 8-IL-8-, leukotriene B4, thromboxane B2) which can damage myelinogenesis in periventricular white matter and lead to periventricular leukomalacia as shown in Figure 2 [Kalis V. et al., 2001; Le Bouar G. et al., 2002; Malamitsi-Puchner A. et al., 2006]. The increased incidence of intrauterine infections in the presence of MSAF, as well as the frequent findings of inflammatory lesions in the placenta, umbilical cord, fetal membranes and lungs, underscores the major role of inflammation in the pathogenesis of fetal brain injury. It is well known that proinflammatory fetal cytokines, oxidants and eicosanoids produce an oxidant environment with deleterious and ischemic effects on fetal neural tissue [Naeye RL., 1995; Wu JM. et al., 1995].

It is however more likely that the etiology of fetal brain injury in cases of in utero meconium passage is synergic. This means that both above mentioned pathogenetic pathways could play an important role in the development of brain damage, but when there is a combination of the two main factors (both direct vasoconstriction on placental vessels and intrauterine infection), then the result becomes more severe. Highly interesting studies are accordingly being carried out based on both the toxic vasoconstrictive role of meconium and the deleterious effects of fetal cytokines and other infection-related factors in the presence of MSAF in order to elucidate the pathogenetic mechanism of fetal brain injury [Benirschke K., 2001].

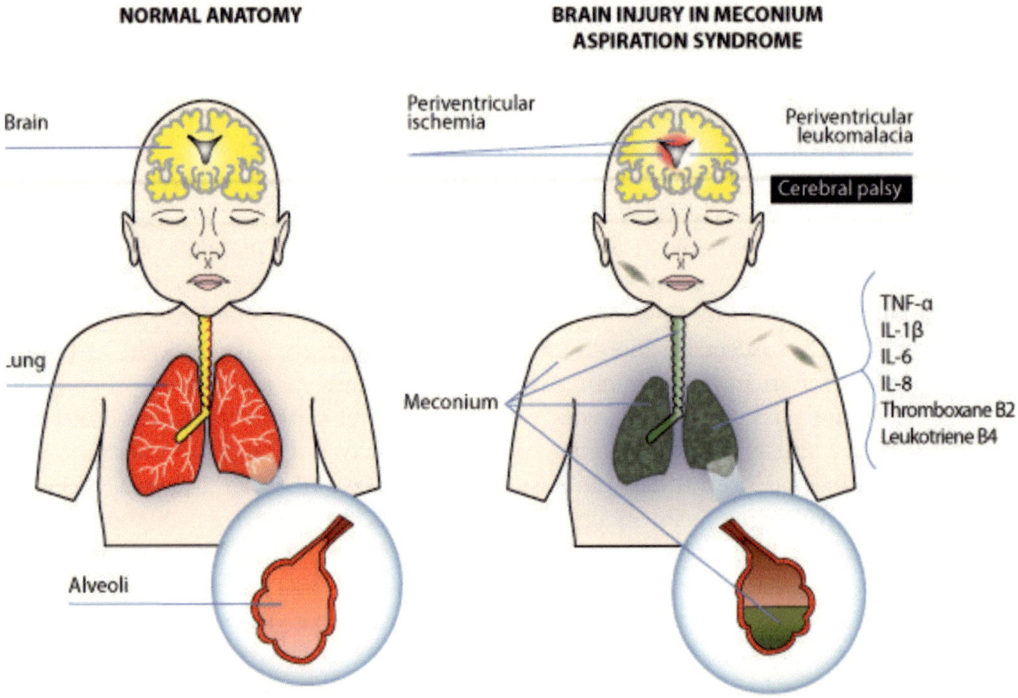

Fig. 2. Pathogenetic pathway of intraamniotic infection due to meconium passage that results in a release of cytokines and eicosanoids from fetal lungs which can damage myelinogenesis and lead to periventricular ischemia and leukomalacia, in comparison with normal neural development in an infant born through clear amniotic fluid without meconium aspiration syndrome.

4. Further neurological abnormalities in children born through MSAF

The vast majority of infants born through MSAF, even after successful management of MAS, do not present symptomatology suggestive of severe neurological disorder due to ante- or intrapartum fetal brain injury. An abnormal fetal heart rate tracing, a low Apgar score in the first and fifth minute after delivery or the presence of recurrent neonatal seizures and symptoms such as hypotonia or lethargy could predict possible CP in future. Nevertheless, even in the absence of these factors during the early postpartum period, an adverse neurodevelopmental outcome, as a result of fetal expose to MSAF, may appear during childhood.

Children born through MSAF present a significantly increased risk for neurologic abnormalities in the 7th year of life, including quadriplegic CP, chronic seizures, hyperactivity, moderate or severe motor disability and severe mental retardation (MR) [Naeye RL., 1992].

Additionally, research studies support the existence of a positive correlation between fetal exposure to MSAF and future development of autistic disorder or difficulty with school learning procedures because of concentration deficit.

In conclusion, it is evident that major neurological disorders may arise from fetal or neonate brain injury. It must be the goal of obstetricians to minimize or even eliminate these complications, so catastrophic for the neurological and mental health of children, and to strive for the best perinatal management and thus outcome for both the mother and the neonate.

5. Conclusions

It is true that most infants born through MSAF will be neurologically healthy. Nonetheless, there is substantial documentation of the existence of a close relationship between MSAF/MAS and development of future neurological abnormalities, as well ample evidence that meconium passage may be the main etiological factor in the pathogenesis of neurological disorders in a significant percentage of children without other obstetrical complications.

The intrauterine environment and the causes giving rise to intraamniotic meconium passage (i.e. hypoxia-anoxia status, intrauterine infection) are also involved in the pathogenesis of fetal brain injury due to MSAF, this possibly being activated via two as yet hypothesized pathways that may act in an either independent or synergic way. The direct vasoconstrictive and/or deleterious long-term in utero effect of meconium results in severe fetal brain injury due to the reduced venous return of oxygenated blood from the placenta to the fetus and/or the environment produced by proinflammatory fetal cytokines, oxidants and eicosanoids which is highly toxic for the fetal neural tissue.

In the vast majority of cases, severe neurologic handicaps do not appear during the early postpartum period. However, the possibly remains that an adverse neurodevelopmental outcome combined with fetal exposure to MSAF could be diagnosed during childhood, or even in the first years of school, translated as pronounced learning difficulties. Cerebral palsy and severe mental retardation are major neurological disorders which are diagnosed more frequently in cases of children born through MSAF in comparison with those born through clear amniotic fluid. Their pathogenetic pathway is likely to have the same origination, which is severe fetal and neonatal brain injury. Needless to say, perinatal care has progressed vastly in the present day and the rate of these complications as well the mortality and morbidity rate after MSAF or MAS are correspondingly much decreased. However, bearing in mind the potential for these adverse outcomes, catastrophic for the neurological and mental future of the child, an uneventful late pregnancy and labor culminating in the optimal perinatal result for both the mother and the neonate must be the goal of every physician.

6. References

Altshuler G, Hyde S. Meconium-induced vasocontraction: a potential cause of cerebral and other fetal hypoperfusion and of poor pregnancy outcome. J Child Neurol 1989;4:137-142

Altshuler G. Placental insights into neurodevelopmental and other childhood diseases. Semin Pediatr Neurol 1995;2:90-99.

Benirschke K. Fetal consequences of amniotic fluid meconium. Contemp Obstet Gynecol 2001;46: 76-83.

Berkus MD, Langer O, Samueloff A, Xenakis EM, Field NT, Ridgway LE. Meconium-stained amniotic fluid: increased risk for adverse neonatal outcome. Gynecol 1994;84:115-120.

Blackwell SC, Moldenhauer J, Hassan SS, Redman ME, Refuerzo JS, Berry SM, Sorokin Y. Meconium aspiration syndrome in term neonates with normal acid-base status at delivery: is it different? Am J Obstet Gynecol 2001;184:1422-1426.

Brews A. Fetal asphyxia. In Eden Hollands Manual of Obstetrics, 9th edn. London: Churchill, 1948:609-612.

Brown CA, Desmond MM, Lindley JE, Moore J. Meconium staining of the amniotic fluid: a marker of fetal hypoxia. Obstet Gynecol 1957;9:91-103.

Cleary GM, Wiswell TE. Meconium-stained amniotic fluid and the meconium aspiration syndrome: an update. Pediatr Clin N Am 1998;45:511-529.

Clifford SH. Clinical significance of yellow staining of the vernix caseosa, skin, nails, and umblinical cord of the newborn. Am J Dis Child 1945;69:327-328.

Fleischer A, Anyaegbunam A, Guidetti D, Randolph G, Merkatz IR. A persistent clinical problem: profile of the term infant with significant respiratory complications. Obstet Gynecol 1992;79:185-190.

Fraser WD, Hofmeyer J, Lede R, Faron G, Alexander S, Goffinet F, Ohisson A, Goulet C, Turcot-Lemay L, Prendiville W, Marcoux S, Laperriere L, Roy C, Petrou S, Xu HR, Wei B, Amnioinfusion Trial Group. Amnioinfusion for the prevention of the meconium aspriration syndrome. N Engl J Med 2004;353:909-917.

Fujikura T, Klionsky B. The significance of meconum staining. Am J Obstet Gynecol 1975; 121:45-50.

Gaffney G, Sellers S, Flavell V, Squier M, Johnson A. Case-control study of intrapartum care, cerebral palsy, and perinatal death. BMJ 1994;308:743-750.

Grafe MR. The correlation of prenatal brain damage with placental pathology. J Neuropathol Exp Neurol 1994;53:407-415.

Kalis V, Turek J, Hudec A, Rokyta Z, Mejchar B. Meconium and postnatal neurologic handicaps. Ceska Gynecol. 2001;66(5):369-377.

Krebs HB, Peters RE, Dunn LJ. Intrapartum fetal heart rate monitoring III. Association of meconium with abnormal fetal heart rate patterns. Am J Obstet Gynecol 1980;137:936-943.

Kuban KCK, Leviton A. Cerebral palsy. N Engl J Med 1994;330:188-195.

Lien JM, Towers CV, Quilligan EJ, de Veciana M, Toohey JS, Morgan MA. Term early-onset neonatal seizures: obstetric characteristics, etiologic classifications, and perinatal care. Obstet Gynecol 1995;85:163-169.

Le Bouar G, Lassel L, Poulain P. Markers of infection and inflammation in the amniotic fluid: Therapeutic contribution of amniocentesis. J Gynecol Obstet Biol Reprod (Paris) 2002;31(7 Suppl):5S52-56.

Malamitsi-Puchner A, Vrachnis N, Samoli E, Baka S, Hassiakos D, Creatsas G. Elevated second trimester amniotic fluid interferon gamma-inducible T-cell alpha chemoattractant concentrations as a possible predictor of preterm birth. J Soc Gynecol Investig. 2006; 13(1):25-29.

Matsuishi T, Yamashita Y, Ohtani Y, Ornitz E, Kuriya N, Murakami Y, Fukuda S, Hashimoto T, Yamashita F. Brief report: incidence of and risk factors for autistic disorder in neonatal intensive care unit survivors. J Autism Dev Disorders 1999;29:161-166.

Mazor M, Hershkovitz R, Bashiri A, Maymon E, Schreiber R, Dukler D, Katz M, Shoham-Vardi I. Meconium stained amniotic fluid in preterm delivery is an independent risk factor for perinatal complications. Eur J Obstet Gynecol Reprod Biol. 1998;81:9-13.

Miller FC, Read JA. Intrapartum assessment of the postdate fetus. Am J Obstet Gynecol 1981;141: 516-520.

Naeye RL. Disorders of the Placenta, Fetus, and Neonate: Diagnosis and Clinical Significance. St.Louis , MO:Mosby Year Book, 1992:257-268, 330-352.

Naeye RL. Can meconium in the amniotic fluid injure the fetal brain? Obstet Gynecol 1995;86(5): 720-724.

Nathan L, Leveno KJ, Carmody TJ, Kelly MA, Sherman ML. Meconium: a 1990s perspective on an old obstetric hazard. Obstet Gynecol 1994;83:329-332.

Nelson KB, Broman SH.Perinatal risk factors in children with serious motor and mental handicaps. Ann Neurol 1977;2:371-377.

Nelson KB. Perspective on the role of perinatal asphyxia in neurologic outcome: its role in developmental deficits in children. CMAJ 1989;141:3-10.

Nelson KB, Ellenberg JH. Obstetric omplications as risk factors for cerebral palsy or seizure Disorders. JAMA 1984;251:1843-1848.

Ramin K, Leveno K, Kelly M. Observations concerning the pathophysiology of meconium aspiration syndrome. Am J Obstet Gynecol 1994;170:312 (#124).

Redline RW. Severe fetal placental vascular lesions in term infants with neurologic impairment. Am J Obstet Gynecol 2005;192:452-457.

Reed CB. Fetal death during labor. Surg Gynecol Obstet 1918;26:545-551.

Sato S, Okumura A, Kato T, Hayakawa F, Kuno K, Watanabe K. Hypoxic ischemic encephalopathy associated with neonatal seizures without other neurological abnormalities. Brain Dev 2003;25:215-219.

Shields JR, Schifrin BS. Perinatal antecedents of cerebral palsy. Obstet Gynecol. 1988;71:899-905.

Spinillo A, Capuzzo E, Stronati M, Ometto A, De Santolo A, Acciano S. Obstetric risk factors for periventricular leukomalacia among preterm infants. Br J Obstet Gynaecol 1998;105:865-871.

Spinillo A, Fazzi E, Capuzzo E, Stronati M, Piazzi G, Ferrari A. Meconium-stained amniotic fluid and risk for cerebral palsy in preterm infants. Obstet Gynecol 1997;90:519-523.

Starks GD. Correlation of meconium stained amniotic fluid, early intrapartum fetal pH, and Apgar scores as predictors of perinatal outcome. Obstet Gynecol 1980;56:604-609.

Steer PJ, Eigbe F, Lissauer TJ, Beard RW. Interrelationships among abnormal cardiotocograms in labor, meconium staining of the amniotic fluid, arterial cord blood pH, and Apgar scores. Obstet Gynecol 1989;74:715-721.

Vain NE, Szyld EG, Prudent LM, Wiswell TE, Aquilar AM, Vivas NI. Oropharyngeal and nasopharyngeal suctioning of meconium-stained neonates before delivery of their shoulders: multicentre, randomized controlled trial. Lancet 2004;364:597-602.

Vrachnis N, Vitoratos N, Iliodromiti Z, Sifakis S, Deligeoroglou E, Creatsas G. Intrauterine inflammation and preterm delivery. Ann N Y Acad Sci. 2010;1205:118-122.

Walker J. Foetal anoxia. J Obstet Gynecol Br Empire 1954;61:162-180.

Wen TW, Eriksen NL, Blanco JD, Graham JM, Oshiro BT, Prieto JA. Association of clinical intra-amniotic infection and meconium. Am J Perinatol 1993;10:438-440.

Wiswell TE, Bent RC. Meconium staining and the meconium aspiration syndrome: unresolved issues. Pediatr Clin N Am 1993;50:955-981.

Wiswell TE, Gannon CM, Jacob J, Goldsmith L, Szyld E, Weiss K, Schutzman D, Cleary GM, Filipov P, Kurlat I, Caballero CL, Abassi S, Spraque D, Oltorf C, Padula M. Delivery room management of the apparently vigorous meconium-stained neonate: results of the multicenter, international collaborative trial. Pediatrics 2000;105:1-7.

Wiswell TE, Tuggle JM, Turner BS. Meconium aspiration syndrome: have we made a difference? Pediatrics 1990;85:715-721.

Woods JR, Glantz JC. Significance of amniotic fluid meconium. In: Creasy RK, Resnik R, editors. Maternal-Fetal Medicine: Principles and Practice. Philadelphia: WB Saunders, 1994;413-422.

Wu JM, Yeh TF, Lin YJ. Increases of leukotriene B4 (LTB4) and D4 (LTD4) and cardio-hemodynamic changes in newborn piglets with meconium aspiration (MAS). Pediatr Res 1995;37:357A

7

Sleep Development and Apnea in Newborns

Adrián Poblano and Reyes Haro
Clinic of Sleep Disorders, School of Medicine,
National University of Mexico and Laboratory of Cognitive Neurophysiology,
National Institute of Rehabilitation, Mexico City,
Mexico

1. Introduction

One of the major problems in neonatal care, is the presence of sleep apnea in premature infants. This is due, that respiratory disturbances placed at high-risk and in immediate danger to newborn infants because alteration in adaptation to extra-uterine environment. Apnea during sleep can be the principal symptom of maturational dysfunction of the control of the central nervous system (CNS) on the infant respiratory patterns, or can be present secondarily to other brain or non-brain pathologies. Frequency of apnea is inversely related to gestational age at birth. In this chapter, we revisited the process of sleep development from fetal to neonatal age focused in the presentation of respiratory alterations, such as the apnea. Afterward, we reviewed the clinical features of apnea for its clinical diagnosis and therapeutics.

2. Development of sleep

Different neuronal networks underlying brain function maturing during fetal life beginning as early as 10 weeks of gestational age (GA). For example, the human fetus displays spontaneous movements that can be visualized by means of ultrasonography (USG), which can document eye-opening and -closure, and rhythmic body movements. On the other hand, fetal heart rate can be electronically recorded by means of serial electrodes placed in the abdominal skin of the mother, fetal heart rate variations reveals the fetal well-being. Both tests, allow estimation of fetal state transitions underlying fetal behavior including the sleep. Recently, Magnetoencephalographic (MEG) recordings of the fetal and neonatal cortical magnetic activity constituted as a promising technique in the study of sleep physiology. At earlier stage of development, no clear sleep state can be well defined. The sleep stages appears clearly at the end of fetal period near at the time of birth.[1] One study carried out in our laboratory suggested a high correlation of fetal sleep with those sleep measurements developed after birth in neonates.[2]

After birth serial recording of several physiologic functions during sleep or polysomnography (PSG) can be obtained by continuous monitoring of electroencephalographic (EEG) signal; eye movements (EOG); electromyographic (EMG) signal of axial and limb muscles; electrocardiographic (EKG) recording; different measurements of respiratory function, such as those obtained by a nasal thermistor, chest and abdominal movements; blood concentrations of oxygen and carbon dioxide sensors are placed in neonates in order to study the organization of the functional state.[3]

Preterm infants born at 24 weeks of gestational age (GA) show predominant cyclic rudimentary sleep functional state called Transitional or Indeterminate sleep (IS). Scarce burst of electro-cortical activity over a flat background in EEG are presents which is called Discontinuous activity or *Tracé Discontinu*.[4] When time intervals are measured between successive epochs of PSG signal, EEG activity shows variable Discontinuous activity depending on GA with larger flat EEG periods at earlier GA. By 34 weeks of conceptional age (CA = GA + post-natal legal age in weeks. Is the better parameter to measure and correct maturational effects of preterm birth and early post-natal life on the EEG and PSG recordings when are compared with those of newborns born at-term and with some weeks of post-natal age) a Rapid eye movements (REM) sleep-like state emerges, and is called Active sleep (AS). Around 37 weeks of CA Quiet sleep (QS) differentiates and appear as alternating intervals of variable span according to CA changes of different EEG frequency and amplitude patterns called *Tracé Alternat*, while in AS periods appears with continuous EEG activity or *Tracé Continu*. Cycle times vary between sleep periods, but usually range between 40 and 60 min. Behavioral estimations of IS approximate amounts 95% of sleep in the 30 weeks of CA studies, decreasing progressively and disappearing by near-term ages.[5]

There is a relative continuity of sleep state from intrauterine through neonatal age, from last weeks of pregnancy to 44 weeks of CA. Such physiologic continuity may reflect the need for sleep state homeostasis of both the fetus and newborn during the transition from intrauterine to extra-uterine environments,[2] requiring approximately one postnatal month of brain development before infant sleep patterns emerge. These physiologic interrelationships defining neonatal state, persist to 4–6 weeks of postnatal life after which infant sleep patterns subsequently emerge to eventually resemble those of adult sleep rhythms by between the first and second years of life. Similar temporal relationships are expressed by preterm neonates in an extra-uterine environment. However, a review of medical literature regarding fetal wakefulness suggests no convincing evidence that the fetus is awake as often as the preterm neonate. A state of cortical arousal similar to IS inhibits the awake state in the fetus as a defense response of brain plasticity.[6]

3. Development of sleep respiratory patterns

The recognition of sleep states in newborns and infants was initially based on differences in respiratory rate. The breathing rhythm was more irregular during AS and IS and more regular during QS segments. Related changes in these respiratory patterns first were noted when sleep state differentiation was recognized.[7] There are a number of features of respiratory patterns that will be briefly summarized, including central respiratory pauses, breathing regularity versus irregularity, breathing frequency, and the percentage of paradoxical breathing as it refers to out-of-phase thoracic and abdominal breathing movements. Central respiratory pauses are of short duration and are normally seen in the newborn and can be documented also during the waking state following body movements. However, they primarily occur during sleep.[8] The apnea index, defined by the percentage of non-breathing time,[9] is significantly higher during AS than QS. It remains high until 38 weeks of CA and decreases significantly both during AS and QS by term age. Preterm infants corrected to term age as well as gestational-age infants who are small for their age also have a greater number of respiratory pauses than is appropriate for gestational-age infants of the same CA.

After 35 weeks of CA, respiratory frequency is higher during AS and QS. During both components of the sleep cycle, respiratory frequency increases with increasing gestational age to term and continues to increase during the first two months of life. Thereafter, at older ages, the respiratory rate progressively decreases. Phase shifting or paradoxical breathing between thoracic and abdominal breathing movements is commonly seen during the first several months of life and is closely related to inter-costal muscle inhibition, particularly during active sleep, in part reflecting high chest wall compliance. By the at-term age of pregnancy, the time spent with 180º out-of-phase shift between thoracic and abdominal breathing movements remains unchanged but is significantly greater during AS than QS.[10]

4. Definition and different types of apnea

Apnea in newborns is defined as absence of breathing for 20 sec or longer, or at a shorter time if bradycardia of <100 beats/min, cyanosis, hypoxia, and/or hypotension is present.[11] Apnea is classified as central, obstructive, and mixed. Central apnea is present when epochs of absence of nasal air flow and thoracic breathing are identified, obstructive apnea is recognized when respiratory thoracic movements are present but nasal air flow is inadequate, and mixed type is present when events begin or end with central or obstructive apnea and change to the other type of apnea.[12] PSG is the most adequate electrophysiologic test to identify apnea in preterm and at-term newborns, and must be performed in all infants with risk factors.

5. Risk factors for different types apnea

We carried-out a study at a tertiary-level medical center for care of high-risk newborns at Neonatal Intensive Care Unit in Mexico City. Newborns were selected if they presented any risk factor for apnea during neonatal period (such as preterm birth, low Apgar score, sepsis, and others) when infants were stable and not mechanically ventilated. The sample was divided in infants that presented and those that did not presented apnea events on PSG studies. Newborns were studied by a neurologic examination, transfontanelar ultrasonography, and laboratory tests. Two hundred twenty three patients were studied (Table 1). One hundred twenty nine were females (57.84%). One hundred thirty one patients were born weighting <1,500 g (58.74%). Apgar score at 1 min was ≤3 in 53 patients, other clinical data were obtained from hospital records.

We detected apnea events in 55 patients (24.66%). Comparison of clinic characteristics between infants with and without apnea is shown in Table 2, significant differences were found with regard to age, weight, and cephalic perimeter at birth, with lower values in the group of infants with apnea as expected by previous literature. No statistical differences in main risk factors such as: sepsis, intraventricular hemorrhage, hyperbilirubinemia, hypoxic-ischemic encephalopathy, meningitis and TORCH in infants with and without apnea were seen. Although each patient can have more than one type of apnea, forty patients showed central apnea events (72.72%), six manifested obstructive events (10.90%), and nineteen demonstrated mixed events (34.54%). Some infants presented only one type of apnea: central (n = 31), obstructive (n = 5) and mixed (n = 10). Comparison of characteristics among these groups showed significant differences in weight at birth, cephalic perimeter, and one-min Apgar score with lower values in infants with central and obstructive apnea than infants with mixed apnea (Table 3). Significant differences in weight at birth between central and mixed groups with regard to infants with obstructive events; and in cephalic perimeter among group of mixed apnea to the other two groups; and in Apgar score at one min in groups of obstructive and mixed apnea to group of infants with central events were observed. Frequency of three main risk factors identified in patients with only one type of apnea showed significant differences when compared with infants without apnea in birthweight <1,500 g in the group of infants with central apnea; and in hyperbilirubinemia and gastroesophagic reflux in infants with obstructive apnea; and in hyperbilirubinemia and sepsis in infants with mixed events of apnea (Table 4). The main pharmacologic agents used for apnea treatment were theophylline (n = 21, 38.18%) and aminophylline (n = 14, 25.45%), nonetheless twenty patients (36.36%) were without treatment at time of study because they were not identified as having apnea events previously.[13]

Risk Factor	*n*	Percentage
Low birth weight (≤ 1,500 g)	131	58.74
Sepsis	120	53.81
Mechanical ventilation	118	52.91
Low Apgar score at minute (≤ 3)	53	23.76
Intracranial hemorrhage	41	18.38
Neonatal seizures	32	14.34
Hypoxic-ischemic encephalopathy	25	11.21
Hydrocephalus	19	8.52
Meningitis	16	7.17
Hyperbilirubinemia (blood exchange)	11	4.93
Cerebral malformation	7	3.13
TORCH	3	1.34
Head trauma	3	1.34

n = number of patients. Each subject can have more than one risk factor

Table 1. Neonatal risk factors in the sample (n = 223 patients)

Variable	Apnea	*x*	*sd*	*p*
Age at birth (weeks)	present	32.82	2.03	0.01
	absent	33.83	3.55	
Weight (g)	present	1405.09	468.44	<0.001
	absent	1738.36	842.88	
CP (cm)	present	28.18	2.58	0.04
	absent	29.16	3.58	
Apgar score 1 m	present	5.56	2.40	n.s.
	absent	6.20	2.36	
Apgar score 5 m	present	8.25	1.17	n.s.
	absent	8.17	1.26	

x = mean. sd = standard deviation. p = probability. n.s. = no significant. CP = Cephalic perimeter

Table 2. Comparison of characteristics of infants with (n = 55) and without apnea (n = 168)

Feature	Type of apnea	x	sd	p
Age at birth (weeks)	Obstructive	32.68	2.23	n.s.
	Mixed	33.76	2.36	
	Central	32.58	2.12	
Weight at birth (g)	Obstructive	1245.09	355.94	0.03
	Mixed	1635.50	421.67	
	Central	1427.41	519.76	
CP (cm)	Obstructive	28.00	2.73	0.04
	Mixed	29.52	2.52	
	Central	28.20	2.70	
Apgar score 1 m	Obstructive	7.2	2.38	0.02
	Mixed	8.00	0.66	
	Central	5.64	2.49	
Apgar score 5 m	Obstructive	8.41	1.34	n.s.
	Mixed	9.00	0	
	Central	7.96	1.35	

x = mean. sd = standard deviation. p = probability. n.s. = no significant. CP = Cephalic perimeter

Table 3. Comparison of characteristic of infants with different type of apnea

Central	n/%	Obstructive	n/%	Mixed	n/%
Preterm birth	30/96.77*	Preterm birth	5/100	Preterm birth	9/90
Sepsis	16/51.61	HB	5/100*	HB	8/80*
HB	13/41.93	GR	3/60*	Sepsis	5/50*
Anemia	12/38.70	HNa	2/40	HM	3/30
HM	11/35.48	IH	2/40		
HNa	9/29.0	BD	2/40		
GR	9/29.03				
BD	8/25.8				
PFC	8/25.8				
FGR	8/25.8				

HB = Hyperbilirubinemia. HM = Hyaline membrane. GR = Gastroesophagic reflux.
HNa = Hyponatremia. IH = Intraventricular hemorrhage. BD = Bronchopulmonar dysplasia.
PFC = Persistent Fetal Circulation FGR = Fetal growth retard. * ($p < 0.001$)

Table 4. Main risk factors found in infants with different type of apnea

6. Pathophysiology

Several mechanisms have been proposed to explain apnea pathophysiology, such as: immaturity of respiratory control center at brainstem, CO_2 lower ventilation response at REM sleep, lower number of synapsis and myelination at respiratory control center.[10,14]

7. Diagnosis and treatment

The diagnosis is clinical, and is established in basis of a high degree of suspicion of apnea in premature high-risk infants. However, some immature at-term infants may also present apnea. Breathing observation and respiratory pauses identification are the cornerstone signs for the diagnosis. However, infants with obstructive and mixed apnea may present some difficulties for the diagnosis. The PSG is the gold standard study for apnea diagnosis of any type because can identify objectively and measure central obstructive and mixed respiratory pauses than can be forgetting by visual observation. Thus, every infants with risk factors or suspicion for apnea must be send to PSG study. Clinical examination must underline in cardio-respiratory and neurological tests. Laboratory studies may include as follows: blood test and culture; lumbar puncture; glycemia and calcium measurements; oxygen and carbon dioxide levels determination; chest, abdominal and gastro-esophagic serial X-ray; echocardiogram; ultrasonography of the brain, and continuous O_2 determination.[15]

For treatment there are several useful interventions: pharmacological and no-pharmacological. We will comment one by one as follows. Methylxanthines increase chemoreceptor sensitivity as well as respiratory drive and can also improve diaphragmatic function. Of the substances available, caffeine has a wider therapeutic range and fewer side effects than theophylline. There were concerns, however, that caffeine, being an adenosine antagonist, could reduce tolerance to hypoxia and might thus be harmful to infants with recurrent hypoxia.[16]

Aminophylline will be given at loading dose of 6-8 mg/Kg and a maintenance dose of 1-3 mg/Kg/dose three times daily to produce a desired plasmatic concentration of 5-12 µg/ml. Theophylline will be given at a loading dose of 7.5 mg/Kg and a maintenance dose of 3 mg/Kg three times daily to produce plasmatic concentrations of 13-20 µg/ml. Caffeine could be administered at a loading dose of 25 mg/Kg caffeine citrate and at a maintenance dose of 6 mg/Kg to produce plasmatic concentrations of 13-20 µg/ml.[17]

Six trials reported on the effect of methylxanthine in the treatment of apnea (three trials of theophylline and three trials of caffeine). Five trials that enrolled a total of 192 preterm infants with apnea evaluated short term outcomes; in these studies, methylxanthine therapy led to a reduction in apnea and use of mechanical ventilation in the first two to seven days. The *post-hoc* analysis of the large Central Apnea of Premature Trial comparing caffeine to control in a subgroup of infants being treated for apnea reported significantly reduced rates of Persistence of Ductus Arterial ligation. Moreover, postmenstrual age at last oxygen treatment, last endotracheal tube use, last positive pressure ventilation; and reduced chronic lung disease at 36 weeks were significantly associated. Methylxanthine was effective in reducing the number of apnea attacks and the use of mechanical ventilation in the two to seven days after starting treatment. Caffeine is also associated with better longer term outcomes.[18]

Other substance used to treat apnea is Doxapram. Doxapram stimulates peripheral chemoreceptors at low, and the central at high doses. It shows a clear dose–response curve, with a 50% reduction in apnea rate occurring in 47, 65, 82 and 89% of infants at a dose of 0.5, 1.5, 2.0 and 2.5 mg/kg/h respectively. Most studies used a continuous intravenous infusion, although some suggest that the i.v. solution may also be given orally at twice the dose with good effect (enteral absorption is approximately 50%). Short-term side effects become quite common at doses above 1.5 mg/ kg / h and include irritability, myoclonus, elevated blood pressure and gastric alterations.[19]

In the other hand, Continuous-positive airway pressure (C-PAP) has been shown to reduce extubation failure in preterm infants, despite the fact that most systems currently available do not reduce work of breathing. C-PAP can be applied via a nasopharyngeal tube or (bi-) nasal prongs. Reintubation rates are 40% lower with the latter device, number needed to treat, which is why this should be the preferred mode when applying C-PAP. An extension to this is Nasal-Intermittent positive pressure ventilation (N-IPPV), which has a high effectiveness over C-PAP in preventing extubation failure. Typically, an inspiratory pressure of 15–20 cm H_2O, applied at a rate of 10–20/min., is combined with a C-PAP level of 5–6 cm H_2O.[20]

Other interventions has been studied such as prone head-elevated positioning, keeping environmental temperature at the lower end of the thermoneutral range, oscillating waterbed and tactile and olfactory stimulation, oxygen administration, increase inspiratory CO_2 concentration, red blood cell transfusions, and branched-chain amino acid supplementation.[16] However, these techniques are under study and deserve more investigation before be accepted.

8. References

[1] Shor Pinsker V, Ugartechea JC, Morales Caballero F, Guzmán Jasso I, López García R, Karchmer S. Characterization of fetal functional states Ginecol Obstet Mex. 1985;53:75-80.

[2] Poblano A, Haro R, Arteaga C. Neurophysiologic measurement of continuity in the sleep of fetuses during the last week of pregnancy and in newborns. Int J Biol Sci. 2007;4:23-8.

[3] Hoppenbrouwers T. Polysomnography in newborns and young infants: sleep architecture. J Clin Neurophysiol. 1992;9:32-47.

[4] Scher MS. Ontogeny of EEG sleep from neonatal through infancy periods. Handb Clin Neurol. 2011;98:111-29.

[5] Poblano A, Garza-Morales S. Usefulness of electroencephalography in evaluation of the newborn. Bol Med Hosp Infant Mex. 1996;53:144-53.

[6] Scher MS, Loparo KA. Neonatal EEG/sleep state analyses: a complex phenotype of developmental neural plasticity. Dev Neurosci. 2009;31:259-75.

[7] Darnall RA, Ariagno RL, Kinney HC. The late preterm infant and the control of breathing, sleep, and brainstem development: a review. Clin Perinatol. 2006;33:883-914.

[8] Curzi-Dascalova L, Christova-Guéorguiéva L, Lebrun F, Firtion G. Respiratory pauses in very low risk prematurely born infants reaching normal term. A comparison to full-term newborns. Neuropediatrics. 1984;15:13-7.

[9] Minowa H, Uchida Y, Ebisu R, Yoshibayashi M, Takahashi Y, Yoshioka A. New desaturation index to evaluate neonatal apnea using polygraphy. Pediatr Int. 2003;45:294-300.

[10] Poets CF. Sleep Med. Apnea of prematurity: What can observational studies tell us about pathophysiology? 2010;11:701-7.

[11] Task Force on Prolonged Apnea. Prolonged apnea. Pediatrics 1978;61:651-2.

[12] Baird TM. Clinical correlates, natural history and outcome of neonatal apnoea. Semin Neonatol 2004;9:205-11.

[13] Poblano A, Marquez A, Hernandez G. Apnea in infants. Indian J Pediatr. 2006;73:1085-8.

[14] Sale SM. Neonatal apnoea. Best Pract Res Clin Anaesthesiol. 2010;24:323-36.
[15] Paul K, Melichar J, Miletín J, Dittrichová J. Differential diagnosis of apneas in preterm infants. Eur J Pediatr. 2009;168:195-201.
[16] Poets CF. Interventions for apnoea of prematurity: a personal view. Acta Paediatr. 2010;99:172-7.
[17] Scanlon JEM, Chin KC, Morgan MEI, Durbin GM, Hale KA, Brown SS. Caffeine of theophylline for neonatal apnea? Arch Dis Child 1992;67:425-8.
[18] Henderson-Smart DJ, De Paoli AG. Methylxanthine treatment for apnoea in preterm infants. Cochrane Database Syst Rev. 2010;12:CD000140.
[19] Yost CS. A new look at the respiratory stimulant doxapram. CNS Drug Rev. 2006;12:236-49.
[20] Campbell DM, Shah PS, Shah V, Kelly EN. Nasal continuous positive airway pressure from high flow cannula versus infant flow for preterm infants. J Perinatol. 2006;26:546-9.